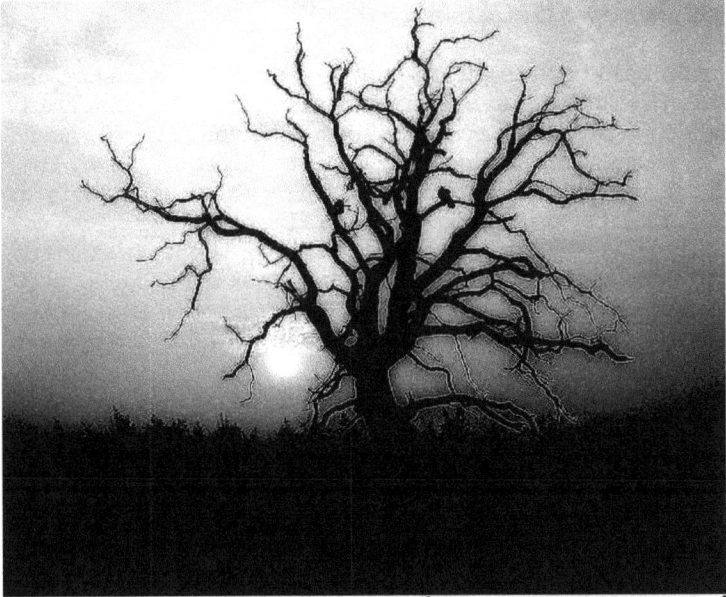

People are trapped in history and history is trapped in them.
James A. Baldwin

Mad! What could be half so horrible?
Nellie Bly, Ten Days in a Madhouse

This story will leave readers torn between rushing to the next page and pausing to savor the author s distinct descriptions and vivid imagery. As a historian, author Sylvia Shults knows how to set the scene, and as an accomplished author, she executes this tale with shocking accuracy and true-to-life realism. This is a fantastic book.
Tamara Thorne & Alistair Cross

44 Years in Darkness is a look back at Rhoda Derry s life, one of the patients at the Peoria State Hospital in Illinois. This book is intended to give the reader a look into the life of one ordinary woman, and how society affected that one life. The author does a brilliant job in detailing the past history of the facility, faculty and history of the times. Shults does a caring and detailed historical job in unearthing the true story of one woman s struggle in a day and age where mental illness was misunderstood and treated. A must read for those interested in history, mental illness and the paranormal as the story continues from beyond the grave.
Alexandra Holzer

Masterful ...I've never read anything that magnetic. The research is top notch. I loved it! (The) writing just flows!
Jerry Ayres, co-host of The Calling

Central Illinois folklorist and author Sylvia Shults has achieved something quite rare in her gripping new historical narrative, 44 YEARS IN DARKNESS -- a terrifying true story rendered with all the heartbreaking emotion of a novel but also steeped in fascinating historical minutiae. The tragic figure of Rhoda Derry is destined to take her place beside all the great mythic martyrs from Lizzy Borden to Joan of Arc. Highly recommended!
Jay Bonansinga

"What a wonderful book! A riveting account of a young woman's descent in to heart-breaking madness that confined her to almshouse hell. Does Rhoda Derry's ghost still drift around her former grounds? Sylvia Shults provides exhaustive historical research and analysis woven into deft storytelling, and lays bare some of her own family secrets as well. There are twists, turns, and surprises in this story from beginning to end.
Rosemary Ellen Guiley

44 YEARS IN DARKNESS

BY SYLVIA SHULTS

A True Story of Madness, Tragedy & Shattered Love

AN AMERICAN HAUNTINGS INK BOOK

Original Cover Artwork Designed by
© Copyright 2016 by April Slaughter & Brandon Thomas Carroll

This Book is Published By:
Whitechapel Press
American Hauntings Ink
Jacksonville, Illinois | 217.791.7859
Visit us on the Internet at http://www.whitechapelpress.com

First Edition – October 2016
ISBN: 978-1-892523-47-1

Printed in the United States of America

CONTENTS

PROLOGUE
TREES IN WINTER

Washington, DC, is hot at the end of June. The sticky heat is just as bad in central Illinois this time of year, though, so he's used to it. It's nothing to get worked up about. Manila was ten times worse in the summer; now he's back home in the United States, so what does he have to complain about?

The Chairman of the Special Committee glances around at the gathered representatives. They are in the House, and the men here are from every state in the Union. It's fitting that the investigation of the Government Hospitals for the Insane is being held in the House of Representatives. Mental illness, too, is well represented in every state in the Union.

The hearings had begun May 4, and they aren't expected to wrap up until the middle of December. He is glad he doesn't have to spend the whole time here. He is already eager to get back to the business of running his asylum.

"The date is June 27, 1906," the chairman says for the benefit of the secretary. "Will you please state your name for the record?"

"Doctor George Anthony Zeller."

"And what is your position, Dr. Zeller?"

"I'm the superintendent of the Illinois Hospital for the Incurable Insane." Dr. Zeller shifts on the hard chair. He really needs to do something about that name. It irks him endlessly, that "Incurable" in the institution's title. No patient is incurable. Desperate, yes. Wretched, perhaps. In need of help, most certainly. But never incurable. He's thought of trying to change the name of the asylum to something a little more innocuous, a little less ... judgmental. Maybe something simply geographical, like ...

"Can you tell us where your asylum is located, Dr.Zeller?"

"It's in Bartonville, Illinois, right on the Illinois River. It's close to the middle of the state, five miles south of Peoria, on the same side of the river. It's 175 miles south and west of Chicago." He likes that accuracy – not "about 200 miles". One hundred and seventy miles from Chicago to Peoria, then another five to Bartonville.

Peoria – that's the closest big town, much larger than Bartonville. Maybe he could get the name changed to Peoria State Hospital. That might lessen the stigma that that infernal word "incurable" always dredges up.

The chairman is talking again, and Dr. Zeller brings his attention back from his asylum, hundreds of miles away in Illinois. He must make a good impression on these Washington bigwigs. It's certain that President Roosevelt – Teddy – will be looking over this report when the investigation wraps up in December. And why not? He and Theodore are kindred spirits. They both care for their fellow human beings on this journey through life. They both have a special place in their heart for children. Dr. Zeller spent a couple of years in the Philippines helping children, and Roosevelt will soon be named president of the American School Hygiene Association.

"The institution having recently been built, I suppose you have the very newest appliances that are known to science in the care of the insane?"

"Yes, sir."

"Science in the care of the insane, like everything else, is advancing, is it not?" The chairman's smile is patronizing.

"That is the idea, sir," Dr. Zeller replies. "In the conduct of our institution we look forward entirely. We had no tradition to govern us, and consequently we took up what we thought was new."

"Have you any pay patients there?"

Dr. Zeller straightens even further in his seat. "I never have accepted pay from any patient since the institution has been going. There is a provision in the Illinois law which allows voluntary pay to the State, but no one ever thinks of offering the State pay for any patient in any State institution, nor would we accept it."

"What is the cost per capita?"

"One hundred and thirty dollars a year net. That includes the entire maintenance of the patients, except for clothing. I think our clothing bill for the past year of nine dollars per capita was rather low, but we contributed to that economy by making a great many of those."

Oh, but this was turning out to be an enjoyable interview after all. The chairman is clearly stunned at the idea that the patients make their own clothes. Scissors? And needles? In the hands of the insane? Unthinkable! The chairman shakes his head in disbelief. "That is, the patients are employed?"

"Yes, sir; a large number of patients are employed, largely in the domestic department."

"What character of patients do you have?"

"We have the worst class of patients that can be found in the nine thousand insane of Illinois." Dr. Zeller can't stop a hint of pride from creeping into his voice. "Our institution is the dumping ground for the other institutions."

"But what is their class?"

Another man speaks up. The nameplate on his desk reads "Mr. Barchfeld" in black letters on the gleaming brass. "They are incurables."

"They are the class that other superintendents choose to send us," Dr. Zeller corrects him.

The chairman turns back to Dr. Zeller. "Do you mean to say that the other institutions of Illinois can send you patients whom you are obliged to receive?"

"Yes, sir. I made a protest about that until it rang all over the State, but they still do it." It isn't that he begrudges being sent these extra patients. He wants to help as many of these poor souls as he can. It's what he does. He just wants to do right by the patients he already has, with the resources he has. "I have received a message just now: 'Will you take one hundred patients from Dunning?' Dunning is the Chicago Insane Asylum. I will answer that: 'Send them along.' When I get those one hundred patients they will be the pick of sixteen hundred insane, and undesirability will be the determining factor in selecting them." A ripple of laughter runs through the room, and Dr. Zeller allows himself a rueful grin at his own expense.

"Is there any particular charter connected with your institution that makes it necessary for you to accept undesirable people from the other insane asylums?" the chairman asks.

Mr. Barchfeld pipes up again. "His is an asylum for incurables."

Dr. Zeller glances at Barchfeld. Why is the man so single-mindedly antagonistic? "My asylum is called the Illinois Asylum for the Incurable Insane," he says, trying to hide his irritation. "There is no law defining incurability in Illinois. It is up to the superintendents."

"Do the newspapers generally jump on your institution?"

"They do not. They stand by me. They are very generous. But please understand me. My institution was built to take from the almshouses of Illinois an accumulated number of incurable insane which had been transferred from the insane asylums to these almshouses. If I were to take those strictly I would get a very nice class of old, demented, quiet patients; but the congestion being so great in the other institutions, the State board of charities has ruled that these other asylums may send their patients to us direct. In the case of Dunning, I am simply relieving Chicago of its burden."

The chairman is really getting involved in his questioning now. "How many attendants and nurses have you in proportion to the number of patients?"

"About one to nine."

"In your opinion have you all the attendants and nurses that are necessary?"

"Yes, sir; I have free choice to select more if I wish them."

"Have you?" The chairman's eyebrow quirks.

Dr. Zeller's nod is brisk, decisive. "No one limits me in the number of attendants."

"What pay do your attendants and nurses get?"

"Every woman in the institution gets twenty dollars. Higher pay depends on promotion. One girl in every five gets a higher position. Each cottage has a head attendant."

"What does she get?"

"Twenty-five dollars. Then we have general night watches, supervisors, and so forth. The corps of graduate nurses get thirty dollars apiece, the supervisors get forty dollars, the matron gets fifty dollars; and all these people are chosen from the mass of attendants." Dr. Zeller is enjoying this recitation so much that he nearly misses the dumbfounded expression on the chairman's face.

"Do you have female attendants altogether?"

"I have one ward that is in the hands of men," he admits cheerfully.

Another man blurts out, "Only one ward?"

"One cottage," Dr. Zeller smiles.

"You have female attendants altogether, do you?" Dr. Zeller is so used to this that it takes him a moment to register the shock in the chairman's voice.

"Yes, sir; over six hundred – nearly seven hundred – of my men are in the care of women attendants."

"How does that operate?" the other man gasps.

"Splendidly." Dr. Zeller doesn't even try to hide the satisfaction in his voice.

"Do you find that the women attendants have difficulty in controlling their people?"

"No, sir."

"You prefer the women attendants for male patients?"

"I certainly do. I regard them as better."

"Why, Doctor?"

Dr. Zeller holds up a hand, folding down fingers one by one as he ticks off his points. "They are better housekeepers. Then we have a homelike atmosphere in the cottage, the presence of a woman about the house. We have also the approval and the gratitude of the visiting friends and relatives of the patients, who universally approve of it."

The chairman has decided to pounce on Dr. Zeller's methods of running the asylum. "Do you lock your wards?"

"No, sir."

"You do not?" The chairman's eyebrows rise. *But they're crazy, and crazy people must be locked away.*

"No, sir."

"The doors of the wards are not locked?"

Why is this so hard for him to grasp? "The doors are not locked and the windows are unguarded."

"And yet you say you only have one attendant to nine patients?"

"That is all, about that; yes, sir." Dr. Zeller allows himself an inward smile, although his face, even at rest, is a study in fierce. It is a point of pride with him, like hiring mostly female attendants, that his wards are left unlocked at all times. He insists, too, that every window be left open about an inch, so that the patients can clearly see that they are not closed in. *These people don't lock their doors at home,* he tells his staff. *Why should we lock them in here, when they've come to us for help?*

The chairman elects to move on. He looks down at his notes. Dr. Zeller's career so far makes for fascinating reading. "How long have you been treating insane people?" the chairman asks.

"Well, I have been actively in charge of this institution since 1902. I was superintendent as early as 1898, but the institution did not open." His wife Sophie sometimes says he has a gift for understatement. The hospital has been plagued with setbacks from the beginning. The dream, conceived by the Bartonville Women's Club, has had its nightmarish moments, including the monstrosity of a Kirkbride building that had to be torn down before one patient even set foot in it. Poor ventilation – and a cracked foundation – wasn't going to do anybody any good, healthy or insane. The colossal waste – a massive building, brand-new, absolutely unfit for human habitation – still made his gut twist. "I was away out of the country."

"Had you had experience with insane institutions before that?"

"No, sir; only such as I had obtained from a study of the subject, from time to time, preparing myself. I was the superintendent, appointed by the governor, a long time before the institution was opened, and pending its completion I was away. It was opened, but I did not get home quite in time for the opening, but I have been continuously the superintendent since October, 1902." How to put such a complicated situation into simple words? How to explain his conflicting duties, his conflicting desires to serve? He wanted to help the insane of Illinois. He'd grown up in that area, swimming in the Illinois River, feeling rich Illinois dirt crumbling between his toes. He loved the area, its productive farmland, the people who worked that land ~ even the people who worked too hard and came down with tuberculosis, or drove themselves into insanity.

But there are the children to think about, too. He remembers the little Filipino children running up to him in the streets of Manila, taking his hands so trustingly. They were never fooled by his serious, unsmiling face, his ramrod posture, his piercing, deep-set eyes, his fiercely bushy mustache. They just knew he made their hurts go away, and they loved him for it.

The chairman turns to Dr. Zeller, looks him up and down. He seems to notice, for the first time, that Dr. Zeller is wearing his dress whites. They're comfortable, especially in the muggy heat of central Illinois. And Zeller is comfortable in the memories the uniform evokes.

"You were in the Army, at Manila, as a surgeon connected with the Army?"

"I was a volunteer surgeon, yes, sir; about three years." Dr. Zeller touches the medal on his chest in an unconscious gesture of reassurance. It is an award given for saving someone's life in the line of duty, and adornment though it is, it is one of his most treasured possessions. During one of the rainy seasons in Luzon, a detachment of colored soldiers was trying to ford a swollen stream. One of the men, Private Cornelius Mitchell, was swept away along with his horse. The rest of the men reached the post, exhausted, and the next morning, Dr. Zeller went out with them to search for Mitchell. They found Mitchell in a native's hut, battered and bruised from his trip down the stream. They brought him back to the post wrapped in blankets, and put him on a cot surrounded by hot water bottles to prevent pneumonia. For his part in the rescue, Captain Charles Young had recommended that Dr. Zeller be given a medal. It had been a recovery, really. Dr. Zeller thought it odd to be the central figure of a drowning in which there was no drowning. Still, he supposed he *had* saved the boy.

It didn't make up for his failure in the very same situation, decades earlier, when a childhood friend lost his life in the Illinois River. That youthful failure, when Zeller was himself just a boy, propelled him into a life in medicine. He wants so desperately to save people – and he does, he reminds himself. He does.

His time in the Philippines is part of that lifelong penance. He agrees with John Hay, the ambassador to the United Kingdom, that the ten months of fighting was "a splendid little war", if such a thing can be said about bloodshed. The Americans who made the trek southward, battling malaria and the Spanish, were sons of Civil War veterans. Whites and blacks both served in a common cause, helping to heal the hurting soul of a country still aching from the fight of brother against brother just a generation earlier. Dr. Zeller is proud to have been a small part of that healing.

Again, Mr. Barchfeld jumps into the conversation. "How many unsuccessful escapes have you had?"

An odd question, but Dr. Zeller is here to answer any questions, no matter how strange. He chuckles. "We have had quite a number of unsuccessful escapes. We think nothing of an escape. If somebody wanders down the hill or off of the grounds there is no fuss. Somebody checks them up and says such and such a patient is missing. Then the hue and cry is raised and we go out and look for him, and in most instances he will be brought in in a reasonable time."

Mr. Barchfeld's eyebrows are nearly part of his hairline. "What do the friends of the patient think of that?"

Dr. Zeller relaxes, and a smile ghosts across his fierce face. "The friends of the patient are our inspiration in all this. They are the people who are sustaining us in this. They like it."

The chairman picks up the questioning. He seems to be searching for any weakness in the asylum's care, and Dr. Zeller is beginning to get a trifle irritated with the fussy little man, although he's careful not to let it show. He understands the man's posturing in front of his peers, the representatives of the United States.

Mental illness is a terrifying thing, and most of these men would rather continue to see the mentally ill as dangerously unbalanced crazies – if they think about them at all.

But Dr. Zeller is here to educate them, to lead them to a different understanding of mental illness – exactly what he hopes to do in Illinois, too. By training his staff to his exacting standards, he hopes to show the world a different face of the severely mentally ill ... the people the rest of the world calls "incurable". And he does that by answering questions, day after day, as patiently as he can.

The chairman glances at his notes. "Take a ward that holds thirty people –"

"We have no such ward," Dr. Zeller says with a trace of smugness.

"What would the ward hold?"

"Sixty is our smallest ward."

"How many attendants do you have on that ward at one time watching those sixty people?"

"Two."

"Do you mean to say that such absolute surveillance can be had by two attendants over sixty patients as to prevent either attacks by patients on attendants or injuries by patients to themselves?"

Dr. Zeller relents. "I'm speaking of a typical ward, where patients are generally on their good behavior."

The chairman huffs irritation. "Then take a case where a ward contains patients who are not on their good behavior."

"Then we have more attendants – probably five on such a ward."

"Let me ask you, then, the question in this way. Granted a ward of disturbed patients, with sixty patients in it, watched by five attendants; can you prevent attacks, or injuries by patients to themselves?"

"It keeps the girls very busy in certain wards," Dr. Zeller says in a dry voice.

One of the representatives – a Mr. Smyser, according to his nameplate – stands, holding a sheaf of papers. He adjusts his glasses on his long nose. "Doctor, I see on page 11 of your report, you say: 'We have a woman who choked two women to death'."

"Yes, sir; we still have her."

" 'And a man who inflicted a fatal bite upon another, and subsequently he killed two women with a fire poker'," Smyser continues.

"Yes, we still have him. I remember him very well."

The chairman can't contain himself. "Do you not think that could have been prevented if they had been restrained?"

Dr. Zeller's reply is calm, measured. "In both cases these things happened in the almshouse before they came to us."

Mr. Hay jumps in again. "You say these things happened –"

"In the almshouse," Dr. Zeller finishes for him. His voice is firm; retirement has not dimmed his military bearing. "I am citing there the character of the patients that are brought to us."

"It did not happen in your institution?" Hay asks.

"No, sir; these people were brought to us after these things had happened."

"Have they hurt anybody since they have been with you?" Hay presses.

Dr. Zeller concedes the point. "Yes, sir; that man bit a man's nose off."

"If you had put that man in mechanical restraint, would that have prevented him biting the nose off?"

Dr. Zeller sighs. "It is a mania with him. He is kept under very close watch now. It is perhaps eighteen months ago that he did that. We had a conversation as to the advisability of pulling the man's teeth, but I could not bring myself to think that the pulling of his teeth would be excused in light of modern ideas in the care of the insane, and the teeth were not extracted. We will take a chance on him not doing it again."

"Will you have to keep him restrained all the time in order to prevent an accident of that kind?" Mr. Hay asks.

"You would have to keep him away from noses," Dr. Zeller shrugs.

Someone in the room barks startled laughter, and Mr. Hay frowns.

Mr. Smyser is still flipping through pages of paperwork. "Doctor, I see on page 12, under the heading 'Curtailments of Restraint' –"

"That is two years old, that report," Dr. Zeller interrupts, fighting the urge to rise from his chair. "I beg your pardon, but please remember that that report is two years old."

"Just a moment. 'Mechanical restraint has been reduced to the minimum, and all other apparatus has been discarded except in a few periodical violent inmates on the male side.' At the time of this writing you did have some sort of restraint?" Mr. Smyser looks up.

"We have abolished the restraint not so very long ago – absolutely abolished it," Dr. Zeller answers. He can't emphasize this enough. It is one of the guiding tenets of the asylum – *his* asylum.

"How recently?"

"On the 25th of September, 1905. That was the day the final order was issued against the use of restraint in our institution. There had been a progressive movement toward its elimination, and it was made final on that day." Dr. Zeller's voice is quiet steel. He loathes any sort of restraint. A nurse must have her hands on a struggling patient, to soothe with a gentle touch. And a human hand can feel the instant of surrender, the instant the struggling stops. Canvas and iron can't *feel.*

The chairman takes up the questioning once more. "When you find patients who seek to injure themselves by picking out their eyes and striking themselves and jabbing things into themselves, what do you do with them?" The chairman is leaning forward, elbows on his desk, waiting, eagerly it seems, for Zeller's answer to this inflammatory question.

And Dr. Zeller himself has been waiting for this very question to be asked. He glances around at the men in the room. Many faces are twisted in polite disgust at the idea that someone could purposefully claw their own eyes out. *My god, that's horrible. Only a crazy person would do that, right?*

But he is prepared for this question. In a way, he has been preparing for this question ever since September 1904. He has been expecting it. And he has a good answer for it. A skeletal, grinning face flashes in his mind's eye. *Rhoda* ... good God, does he ever have a good answer.

"We have a patient who was forty-four years in an almshouse who plucked out both eyes in her madness," he says. He tries to ignore the whisper of revulsion that rushes through the room like a fetid breeze. This is Rhoda's story, and it is important, and he will tell it. "She has been with us a couple of years now."

The chairman can't hide the horrified fascination in his voice. "Did she pluck out her eyes in the almshouse or after she came to you?"

"She did it in the almshouse."

"That is what you call suicidal mania, is it not?"

Dr. Zeller frowns in irritation. "Yes, you might call that suicidal." But in truth, he has never seen a patient with a stronger will to live. In spite of her appalling circumstances, Rhoda is alive.

Rhoda, her sightless, skeletal face still before him, is one of the reasons he is here in Washington DC, testifying before the Special Committee on Investigation of the Government Hospital for the Insane. She is one of several hundred reasons, really, the reasons currently wandering the grounds of the Illinois Hospital for the Incurable Insane, or shivering in the beds of the wards, watched over by attentive nurses.

"Trees in winter," he murmurs to himself, far too softly for the secretary to pick it up, far below the hearing of the aggressive chairman. It's a reminder to himself.

That morning, as he was standing in front of the hotel room mirror, settling his cover, Sophie had come up behind him. She had brushed an invisible speck of dust from his shoulder, letting her small hand rest there for a moment.

"Remember the trees in winter," she had said, and Dr. Zeller had nodded in understanding. It has been a private code between them for years, a way to explain their devotion to the patients in their care.

Dr. George Zeller, and Sophie too, sees the mentally ill, the demented, those with nowhere else to turn, as trees in winter. They may be stark, gaunt, skeletal. They may look like they have little or nothing to offer. They may not be useful, or beautiful, or productive in any real sense of the word. But they deserve care and unconditional love just like any other human being.

They are alive, just like trees in winter.

PART ONE: THE BEGINNING

CHAPTER ONE
RHODA DERRY

The story of Rhoda Derry is one of the great tragedies of mental health care in Illinois, and one of the great triumphs of the Peoria State Hospital. The old phrase "truth is stranger than fiction" seems to have been made up just to describe the story of Rhoda's life ... and quite possibly, her afterlife.

Rhoda was born in Indiana in 1834, the youngest of nine children. Her family moved to Lima, Illinois, near Quincy in the western part of the state, when Rhoda was still just a child. She grew up there, blossoming into a legendary beauty. In different circumstances, Rhoda would have lived an ordinary life. She would have had children. She would have died peacefully, and been remembered decades later by a descendant flipping through an old photo album. She would have been captured in a wedding tintype, perhaps, sitting posed elegantly with a bouquet while her new husband stood behind her. "Wow, look at how pretty Great-grandma Rhoda was," a child would say, and turn the stiff black page. Rhoda might never have had any notoriety, never been known beyond the private history of her own family, never been a source of fascination to anyone other than the genealogists of her own descent – but she made one fatal mistake.

She fell in love.

She spent the rest of her life paying for that mistake. In a few short years, she went from blissfully happy to utterly miserable. Rhoda ended up confined in the Adams County almshouse for decades. She would have died there, an anonymous tragedy, a shameful family secret spoken of in hushed tones if at all ... but miraculously, she was rescued.

In 1902, more than forty years after Rhoda was committed to an almshouse, the Illinois Asylum for the Incurable Insane opened its doors to the lunatic population of the state. It was located in Bartonville, on a bluff top overlooking the Illinois River. The Women's Club of Bartonville founded the asylum, and chose for their superintendent Dr. George A. Zeller, a respected physician. Dr. Zeller made it his business to visit the almshouses around the state, and to rescue the most pathetic, abused, wretched cases and bring them to his modern, state-funded, state of the art institution. Dr. Zeller found Rhoda. He took her into his care.

He saved her.

Rhoda Derry became famous during the last two years of her life. Her case was so astonishing that reporters and other visitors to the asylum couldn't help but be fascinated by her story. Dr. Zeller and his protective nurses never let Rhoda become an object of curiosity. Instead, they used her case to gently remind reporters, politicians, and other influential people that the asylum was doing real good for its patients.

Rhoda died in 1906, but her story continues to resonate through the years. In 2010, an indie film company called Reality's End began work on a movie about Rhoda's life. Their experiences making that film convinced them there was more, much more to Rhoda's story. And tales of Rhoda's spirit add to the wealth of ghost stories surrounding the Peoria State Hospital, one of the most haunted places in the United States.

This book is a look back at Rhoda's life, and the events that led to her forty-plus-year incarceration in an almshouse. It's also an examination of the supernatural activity that still goes on at the Peoria State Hospital – activity that includes Rhoda.

I first heard Rhoda's story years ago, when I was writing my first collection of true ghost stories. I later wrote a book dealing with the hauntings at the abandoned asylum. In researching *Fractured Spirits: Hauntings at the Peoria State Hospital,* I stood at Rhoda's grave many times. I read a book written by Rhoda's great-grand-nephew, D. Doc Derry.

And the more I learned about Rhoda's story, the weirder it got.

There is a single photograph that is said to be an image of Rhoda Derry, taken at the end of her life. The figure in that picture is a wizened mummy, grinning toothlessly at someone behind the photographer, her knuckles swollen from years of using her hands as feet. She sits on the floor because she can no longer sit in a chair. She is a grotesque caricature of a human being, like something out of a nightmare. This is the image most people have of Rhoda – this is the image that shows up on Pinterest, of all places, when Google is asked to find information on Rhoda Derry.

But Rhoda didn't always look like that. She was once a gorgeous young lady, poor, but pretty enough to catch the eye of a well-to-do farmer's son. She laughed, lived, loved. I wanted to show Rhoda Derry in all her variety, not just the hollow shell she became.

This book is intended to give the reader a look into the life of one ordinary woman, and a look at the society that shaped her. I have taken a few dramatic liberties with Rhoda's story, imagining scenes between her and her intended, Charles Phenix. But the facts of Rhoda's life and history are so compelling, there's really no need for embellishment beyond simply setting the scene.

The story of Rhoda Derry, as strange and terrifying and touching as it is, is not a work of fiction.

It's true. It really happened. This is a story of young love, of bitter loss, of mental illness, of abandonment and redemption, a story given to us by history itself.

And it started with a kiss.

CHAPTER TWO
EARLY ILLINOIS

Both small towns of Lima and Ursa, Illinois, lay in the massive chunk of western Illinois known as the Military Tract. This was land owned by the United States government, which had taken it from the Sauk tribe. The Sauk, long-time trading partners with the British, fought the Americans during the War of 1812 when the Americans attempted to take control of the territory along the Mississippi River. In 1813, the Sauk migrated into Missouri, and in 1816, western Illinois officially became part of the United States when the Potawatomi tribe ceded six million acres of Illinois territory. In 1815, surveyors from the General Land Office began marking out the boundaries of the 87,000 square mile wedge of land between the Illinois and Mississippi Rivers.

In return for their service, veterans of the War of 1812 were entitled to a hundred and sixty acres in the Military Tract. Of the territory's 5,360,000 acres, two-thirds were reserved for soldiers' bounties. Each soldier received a deed to his parcel. The mail system was dodgy in those days, so many of the men who came to the area were surveyors and land agents, tasked with making sense of who actually owned which parcel of land. Many of the soldiers, though, were disinclined to farm the land on the western frontier. Some unfortunate Yankees came out to take possession of their land, then found out that farming was a much different proposition than soldiering. Quite a few men found that they had spent all their money getting to their land in Illinois, then had no idea how to go about farming it – and were dead broke. Land speculators would buy up these tracts from the hapless soldiers, giving them enough capital to make their way home, back East. During the 1830s, those speculators sold a lot of the land to farmers who would settle there and start farms.

Illinois is considered a northern state now, but when Rhoda and Charles were born, the state had a decidedly Southern accent. In 1818, when Illinois was granted statehood, it had a population of around 35,000. Of those, four out of every six residents of Illinois were of southern origin. There were three main groups of people who came to settle in the Military Tract; New Englanders, folks from the mid-Atlantic states, and Southerners. The Yankees tended to see the southern immigrants as hopelessly backwards, even ignorant. The Southerners, for their part, thought the Yankees put on airs and were condescending to them. To be fair, they weren't wrong. The Yankees of Illinois went so far as to refer to poor white Southerners as "white folks", to distinguish them from blacks.

We also think of Illinois as being a slave-free state in the years before the Civil War. This, too, was not exactly the case. When Illinois became a state in 1818, it was, on paper, free of slavery. But many of the settlers of the time were French, and they did own slaves. So the Illinois Constitution of 1818 protected slavery in some cases, and allowed Southern slave owners to bring blacks into the state for specific purposes. Slavery didn't become illegal in Illinois until 1848.

Illinois law even made things difficult for slave owners who wanted to free their slaves. They were required to stand for the good character of the blacks, and if the newly freed slaves became a burden on the state, their former owners were responsible for their upkeep.

The opening of the land office in Quincy in February 1831 touched off a wave of migration to western Illinois. With government prices of Military Tract land at $1.25 an acre, people flocked to the area. For several centuries, the Native Americans had been benefitting from the proximity of two of the great rivers of Illinois. Part of the fur trade between the Europeans and the Indians involved shipping furs (deer, muskrat, raccoon, beaver, otter, and bear) from St. Louis to Pittsburgh on the Ohio River. Guidebooks for settlers headed to Illinois touted the advantages of buying land in the Military Tract: cheap land, fertile soil, and convenient river and railway connections to markets.

The Panic of 1837 put the brakes on land sales, but settlers were allowed to occupy the land and cultivate it, if they ponied up the money for a tax lien on land that was in delinquent status. Of course, with land prices so low, anyone with $200 to spare could buy a parcel of timber and prairie and start up a farm.

The geography of western Illinois was ideal for settlement. The wooded areas were mostly burr oak, black oak, hickory, and butternut. These nut trees provided plentiful foraging for the hogs that were allowed to roam the forest. The woods also provided game – deer, turkey, rabbit, and quail – to supplement settlers' diets. The prairie was crisscrossed with creeks and streams – a lucky break. Nobody wanted to dig a well through tough prairie sod. A stream could also provide power for a lumber or flour mill. The year 1849 was the farming year examined in the 1850 census. In 1849, Adams County was one of the biggest producers of wheat in Illinois, providing between three and five bushels per improved acre. By the 1840s, wheat surpluses in the Military Tract were so far above local needs that the excess was shipped to market.

Add to this the ease of getting products to market on the Mississippi and Illinois Rivers, and on the railroads that soon stitched their way across the landscape, and the Illinois Military Tract had a lot of appeal to settlers in the first half of the nineteenth century. The economic possibilities were a powerful draw, but guidebooks of the time plucked at the strings of family devotion as well.

The aim of these guidebooks was to lure farmers into settling down in the Military Tract, and the writers weren't above using a bit of emotional blackmail. One guidebook writer warned that if his readers weren't able to provide land for their sons, "they must then be turned out into the world, and trust to the winds and waves of fortune, which may waft them on to competency and virtue, and which may bear them away to utter and hopeless poverty and irreclaimable vice". The choice was clear: if they stayed in the East, their sons could be lost to cesspools of vice and poverty, but if they moved out to Illinois, their children would be nearby, well-provided for, and would eventually inherit their parents' legacy.

Lima Township is in the northwest corner of Adams County. The western part of the township was originally swampland, saturated from time to time by overflow from the Mississippi River which flowed on the western border of the township. This slough was known as Lima Lake, and some of the best fishing and hunting in western Illinois was to be found there.

Not all of the hunting done around Lima Lake was recreational, though. Sometimes the farmers of the area would go out to cut down on the pest population of the countryside. During one of these hunts, in 1833, it was said that on Bull's branch, hunters discovered a snake den with a hundred and eighty snakes writhing together. When the settlers were first breaking the prairie sod, they would tell of killing twenty to thirty rattlesnakes a day. They would set fire to the grass to make the sod easier to cut. The fire would drive the snakes out of the tall grass. A writer of the time helpfully described the difference between timber rattlesnakes and prairie rattlesnakes: timber rattlers were four feet long, with bright copper spots, which made them easy to see in the grass. Prairie rattlers, on the other hand, were smaller and dirt-colored, and harder to spot.

One mile east of the town of Lima was the White Oak branch of the lake, which circled around and eventually emptied into Bear Creek. Further west of White Oak branch was a rough patch of wilderness known as Pea Ridge. The wild country was far from worthless, even in its untamed state. The forests on Pea Ridge were high-quality white oak, and when those trees were harvested for manufacturing purposes, the land they had been dominating proved to be ideal for growing wheat, another cash crop.

It was the German settlers in the area, though, who put the land to even better use – they planted grapevines and started producing wine, in a nod to their Rhineland heritage. The land directly around the village of Lima was especially suited for fruit culture, in particular the cultivation of apples. Lima ranked first in the county in apple growing. The plateau formed by White Oak branch on the east and Lima Lake on the west was some of the richest farmland in the state of Illinois, turning out amazing quantities of corn, wheat, oats, apples, and other staple products. And in the center of the plateau was the little town of Lima.

In 1833, Dr. Joseph Orr built the first general store in the area. The fact that a store was there pretty much guaranteed a town would spring up around it. Dr. Orr was, at the time, playing host to a friend visiting from Peru. The Peruvian declared that he had been to many countries in his travels, but that nowhere had such beautiful women as the capital of his native country. However, he noted gallantly, the women in this new town ran a very close second. He therefore suggested to Dr. Orr that they call the new town Lima. (Of course, the inhabitants continued the southern Illinois habit of using a completely different pronunciation than the namesake city. Hence we get "KAY-ro" for Cairo, "VY-enna" for Vienna, New BER-lin instead of New Ber-LIN, and Lima, which is pronounced LYE-ma like the bean, not LEE-ma like the capital of Peru.)

A town named for the beauty of its female inhabitants – what a perfect place for Rhoda Derry to grow up. According to family legend, Rhoda was a strikingly beautiful young woman in 1850, when she met Charles Phenix. A strong, trim teenage girl with long dark hair, she would definitely have caught the eye of another healthy teenager. D. Doc Derry, Rhoda's great-great nephew, wrote, "Personally, that doesn't surprise me. After all, Derry women are beautiful, and I can attest to that fact when thinking about my daughter, granddaughter, and nieces."

Rhoda was born in Fayette County, Indiana, on October 10, 1834, the youngest of the nine children of Jacob and Rachel (Bright) Derry. The family started off in Pennsylvania and worked their way steadily westward, finally settling in Lima.

Rhoda and Charles were sixteen when they met, but their backgrounds could hardly have been more different. The Phenixes, Frederick and Nancy, were a well-off farming family. Charles was one of four children born to the prosperous Frederick and Nancy.

The Derrys, on the other hand, were quite poor. Jacob Derry was never quite able to make a go of farming, even in the fertile plateau where Lima was located. In fact, many of the references to the Derrys in various census records show them living not on their own farm, but in other people's houses.

Rhoda was the youngest of the Derrys' nine children – the baby of the family. It's possible that, as much as they were able given their reduced circumstances, her parents spoiled her. This is pure conjecture, of course, but a young girl with Rhoda's looks, the youngest child, could grow up with a firm idea of what she wanted.

And what Rhoda wanted, at age sixteen, was Charles Phenix.

Ursa Township is the largest township in Adams County. In 1830, a merchant named Peter Vannerst built the first frame building in "Old Ursa". Vannerst also served as the first postmaster when Richard M. Johnson established the post office. The fact that it had its own post office notwithstanding, Old Ursa was never officially designated as a village. "New Ursa" was founded in 1875, less than a mile north from the Ursa Charles Phenix would have known. In 1875 William B. Smith sold off acre parcels at the crossing of the public road and the railroad branch. Shops and private residences soon sprang up where the Quincy and Warsaw public road and the C., B., & Q. Railroad intersected.

Ursa's role in commerce was also bolstered by its location just seven miles east of the Mississippi River. The countryside around Ursa was honeycombed with numerous springs and several creeks, including Bear Creek, which wandered down from the north after curling around Lima.

The land around Ursa was just as fertile as the country around Lima. The focus just to the south was not so much on wheat as it was on livestock, especially the raising of dairy cows.

Charles wasn't born in Ursa. He was a transplant, just like Rhoda. He was born in Kentucky, as were his parents, Frederick and Nancy, and his older sister Elizabeth. The family moved to Illinois around 1836, before Charles' younger two siblings were born. So they'd been in the state for about fourteen years when Charles and Rhoda met.

Fourteen years is long enough, when you're living in a small town, to settle in, to gain a reputation for yourself. The Phenix family seems to have been well-off, and well-respected. Even Charles, as young as he was, appears to have been known as a level-headed youngster. How do we know this? It's a bit of guesswork, true, but we do know that when Charles was only thirteen years old, he was called into court, along with his father, Frederick – as a witness in an "assault to kill" case.

The court system in western Illinois at that time was used mostly for settling debts – usually less than $100, but many of $80 or $90. The threat of being embarrassed by a public trial was an effective way to keep people current on their financial obligations. These trials were open to the public, and often provided a bit of entertainment for farmers who were willing to take a Saturday afternoon off and take a wagon ride into town.

However, the courts were also used for settling violent disputes. The countryside may have seemed quiet when compared to cities of the nineteenth century, but the peaceful landscape often hid complicated relationships. As one writer put it, "In the unfenced open country, where guns were handy for hunting and farm tools had sharp points, an argument over a stray cow could quickly become assault."

In the fall of 1847, one of these simmering feuds boiled over into violence. According to court records, on October 20, 1847, the court heard a case between Edmund Martin, the defendant, and William B. Martin, the complainant. (It's not explained in the records if the two men were related, but in a small town, it's a safe bet they were.) Edmund Martin came under indictment by the Grand Jury of the County for "the crime of making an assault with the intent to commit murder". On September 1, 1847, Edmund loaded a gun and held it on William.

The faded, spidery writing of the records tells an intriguing story. William went to Edmund's house with several other men, including Frederick and Charles Phenix. While there, William told one of the witnesses not to buy fruit from Edmund until after another of the witnesses had gotten there – there seemed to be an argument over price, because William said "they intended to have it whether the defendant [Edmund] was willing or not", and then they could get it cheaper. Edmund asked to borrow a pistol from one of the witnesses – then he loaded it and pointed it at William, threatening to shoot him.

Edmund didn't ask for a continuance at his trial. He basically admitted that the witnesses were correct, and he was willing to take his punishment, whatever it was. Bail was set at $1000. (It's frustrating that none of the witnesses were named in the court records – it would be interesting to know who said what, especially if either Frederick or Charles were involved more than tangentially in the argument.)

This was still the frontier, of course. But I do find it intriguing that the word of a thirteen-year-old boy held just as much weight in court as that of his father. Charles must have been quite a remarkable young man.

CHAPTER THREE
THE DERRY FAMILY

Of the Derry's nine children, the oldest – Philip, Basil, and Carlisle – were out of the house by 1843. Philip and Basil married and lived in Illinois with their wives, and Carlisle stayed in Indiana, then married and moved to Missouri with his bride. Oldest sister Mary Jane married Anderson Slater – her brother-in-law, older brother to Basil's wife Sallie Slater.

With nine children in the family, each sibling had to make their own way in the world. Each child had to work to make a name for himself – or herself. Philip, the oldest, tried to do this in a big way. He married Cynthia Pribble in 1841, and they lived in Adams County for a while, welcoming their first two children (Jacob, born October 1, 1846, and Edna D. "America" Derry, born October 17, 1849).

Around that time, news began to come from the west – gold had been discovered, and folks were flocking to California and Oregon. The lure of gold was too powerful to resist, so in 1850, Philip gave his brother Basil power of attorney over his affairs. And in the summer of 1851, Philip and Cynthia packed up their belongings, gathered their two small children, and set off to seek their fortune. They were one of the first families to travel to Oregon via the Barlow Route, crossing over Mount Hood.

It was a daring move. Cynthia was pregnant with the couple's third child during their travels across the Great Plains and over the Rocky Mountains. But the little family arrived safely in Oregon City in Oregon Territory before the first snowfall. Basil Bois Derry was born March 22, 1852. Basil was just barely two months old when the family was on the move again, this time south to Jacksonville. Philip was taking the family to the mining camps, to finally begin their search for gold.

Then, tragedy struck. Philip and Cynthia were traveling by horseback – the only good way to get from Oregon City to Jacksonville. The trail led through a canyon, and the riders had to follow a creek bed for most of the way. Cynthia's horse lost its footing on the slippery stones of the creek bed, and Cynthia broke her arm in the fall. The break went bad, and three months later, Cynthia Derry was dead.

While she lay ill, a woman named Jane Wright came to care for Cynthia and baby Basil. After Cynthia's death, on October 10, 1852, the Wrights continued to care for the infant.

But fate and tragedy weren't yet finished with the young family. The next year, in the spring of 1854, Philip fell ill. He wrote out a will on March 20, 1854. Nine days later, on March 29, he died at the home of Towner Savage.

Although Philip's will requested that his three orphaned children stay with Towner Savage, only the oldest, Jacob, actually did. Edna was adopted by the family of Reverend Obed Dickinson, and eventually took their family name. Baby Basil stayed with Jane and William Wright.

Brother Basil's story was just as fraught with drama, but it had a happier ending. Basil married Sarah (Sallie) Slater around 1841. They spent ten years together, and had five children – Sarah Catherine, Rachel Jane, Nancy Elizabeth, Carlisle, and William. Then, in 1851, Sallie, Carlisle, and William all died.

William was the first to go. He was about six weeks old when he died in March. Then, his brother Carlisle died in June. He was not quite three years old. Six months later, mother Sallie passed away. Derry family historian Doc Derry has found no explanation for this series of tragic events. According to his research, there was no epidemic going on in the Quincy area at that time. Maybe all three died from a disease, from cholera or smallpox or typhoid fever. (The three older daughters, and Basil, were fine.) Maybe there were three different causes of death. Maybe it was just plain bad luck for the young family.

Basil married again in May 1852, just five months after Sallie's death. His new bride, Fredericka Christena Weidenheimer, was a young widow – she had married John Niebuhr in 1847, but he had died March 1848. At the time of his death, Fredericka was only nineteen years old. She was twenty-three when she married Basil. Basil and Fredericka went on to have seven children together.

Basil also fought in the Civil War, serving with the 84th Illinois Infantry Regiment. The regiment was organized at Quincy in August 1862, and fought at Chickamauga and Kenesaw Mountain. The regiment participated in the Atlanta campaign, and fought battles at Franklin, Nashville, and on Lookout Mountain with Hooker's division.

Basil served in this unit alongside his brother-in-law, John Jacob Weidenheimer. Also serving along with Basil and John was William Alexander, Basil's son-in-law. The only action Basil saw was the battle of Stones River, Tennessee, on December 31, 1862, and possibly again on January 2, 1863. He must have been wounded in the battle, as he was discharged January 4, 1863, at Bowling Green, Kentucky, for disability. Basil left the army and came safely home. He became a United Brethren minister, and died March 14, 1899. Fredericka lived until September 5, 1903.

There were more Derry siblings, but their deeds have mostly been lost to time. They were farmers – James McCann Derry was still farming in his seventies, living in Missouri, in 1906. The girls grew up to be farmers' wives. All of them ... except for Rhoda.

CHAPTER FOUR
THE MEETING

It is a beautiful spring day in 1850. Rhoda Derry blows a stray strand of dark hair out of her eyes with an impatient puff. It isn't that she minds going to things like a barn raising. She enjoys the chance to socialize, and at sixteen years old, visiting is a welcome change from the boring daily trudge of farm life.

But, she thinks as she stands next to her mother behind the long trestle table, a spring afternoon like this is made for wandering in the woods hunting mushrooms, not waiting to serve sweaty men who'd just spent the day knocking together a barn. Yes, she is looking forward to the barn dance that evening. There are sure to be some good-looking boys there to dance with. But still, she chafes. Oh, she is proud to have contributed to the dinner. Her bread is the finest in the county, she is sure, and her oatmeal pie can't be beat.

She can't shake the glum feeling, though, that the only reason her family has been invited to help with this barn raising was that the Derrys are known to be hard workers. She sniffs to herself. And what has hard work ever gotten them? Not much, that was for sure. The Derrys are still dirt poor. She'd bet they are probably the poorest folks in Lima. She frowns and thrusts the spoon savagely into the bowl of buttered corn.

"Hey, what'd that corn ever do to you?"

The voice is smooth as sorghum molasses. Rhoda looks up into the most beautiful slate-gray eyes she has ever seen.

"Oh ... nothing," she stammers, suddenly shy. "Did you – were you helping to raise the barn?"

"All day," the boy grins, and Rhoda could kick herself for the sheer idiocy of the question. "Funny, though. I don't think I've seen you before now. I'd have remembered." He smiles, and Rhoda's knees go weak.

"You must be hungry after all that work," she says, finding her smile. "Can I get you anything?"

"Plate of food would be good." Again, that cheeky grin.

"How 'bout you find a seat, and I'll bring it to you. I don't mind." Rhoda hears the words tumble from her mouth, and finds, to her astonishment, that she means them. The boy looks to be about her own age. He doesn't live in Lima – she'd have noticed him if he did. She has to find out more about him.

The boy nods and turns away. Rhoda watches him go – just to note where he sits, she tells herself. As soon as he pulls out a chair at a nearby table and plumps wearily into it, she busies herself fixing a plate.

He's been working all day, he's probably famished … a piece of fried chicken … and who doesn't like a good slice of ham? Now Rhoda dithers as she casts her gaze on the serving bowls crowding the table. Corn bread, that's good … oh, supposing he doesn't like green beans?

Finally the plate is full. Rhoda stops to grab a mug of lemonade, and carries them both to the table where the boy sits. He stands as she approaches, which makes her feel like a real lady. She puts the plate down in front of him.

"That looks real good," the boy says. "I'm Charles, by the way. Charles Phenix. This here's my folks." He gestures to an older couple, a teenage girl, and two younger kids, a boy and a girl.

"Happy to meet you. I'm Rhoda Derry." Rhoda ducks her head at the Phenixes. To Charles, she says, "Hope you enjoy the food. And the lemonade." She gives him her brightest smile.

"There's a big slice of oatmeal pie with your name on it waitin' for you when you're done. I made it myself." Rhoda thinks she sees a disapproving frown ghost its way across Mrs. Phenix's face, but she ignores it. "So come on up whenever you're ready."

"Oh, I'll be back, don't you worry. I wouldn't miss your pie for anything." Charles smiles and turns to his plate.

"So, how did you two meet?" It's easy dinner-party conversation, a way to break the ice over cocktails and appetizers. And at an engagement party or a wedding, it gives the star couple a chance to coo over each other in the spotlight without looking like complete soppy idiots.

The truth is, we have no idea how Rhoda Derry and Charles Phenix met. They could easily have met at a barn raising. They both lived in small towns in Adams County, Illinois. The two communities of Lima and Ursa were less than ten miles apart, and it's likely the two small farming towns pooled their resources for communal events.

Charles and Rhoda could also have met at something more celebratory, less utilitarian than a barn raising. County farm societies in Illinois started to sponsor agricultural exhibitions as early as the 1820s, and these fairs were still going strong during the 1840s. In the early 1850s, the state legislature established agricultural societies charged with overseeing the work of county groups. These state-level groups were also responsible for organizing state fairs. Adams County was in a very agrarian part of Illinois. Agricultural exhibitions, and later, state fairs, served a purpose beyond allowing farm families a chance to get off of the homestead and socialize. They also served as clearinghouses of information and places to exchange ideas and pick up new farming techniques. As prosperous farmers, Frederick Phenix and his son Charles may have eagerly looked forward to these gatherings.

Farmers got help in running their homesteads from a variety of sources, but by far the biggest source of cheap labor was one's own family. Illinois farmers raised hogs for their own use, and to sell at market. They kept cows, and farm wives turned the milk into butter and cheese. By the age of ten, at the very least, a farm boy was helping his father in the fields. By the age of fifteen or so, he was doing a man's work. Most fathers didn't pay their sons any wages. In fact, if a teenage son earned wages elsewhere, that money was expected to be turned over to the patriarch. In return, though, sons could expect their father to help them acquire their own farms when they came of age and got married.

As one of only two sons in the family, Charles Phenix could look forward to a comfortable inheritance, enough to set him and a wife up on a farm of their own. This was probably a big source of friction between his mother, Nancy Phenix, and Rhoda Derry.

And what about the role Rhoda was supposed to play in the household economy? As poor as the Derrys were, they (or the families they boarded with) would probably have had a cow. They kept chickens for meat and eggs. Sheep provided wool, which was spun into yarn, again by the women in the household. By the middle of the nineteenth century, only some of this yarn was being knitted or woven into clothing for the family's use. More often, it too was sold.

Candlemaking was another task of frontier households, and a very tedious job it was. There were molds that could produce six, twelve, or even twenty-four candles at a time, but most candles were formed by dipping the wicks in beef or deer tallow. It took three or four hours of dipping, putting on one thin layer of tallow at a time, to make six candles. And a house of average size might use three dozen candles a week. Christiana Holmes Tillson, in her book *A Woman's Story of Pioneer Illinois*, writes of dipping sixteen dozen candles in the fall and twenty dozen in the spring. The tallow for the spring batch had to be boiled in alum water to harden it for use in the summer.

F.M.Perryman, author of *Pioneer Life in Illinois*, wrote that there was little difference on the frontier between men's and women's work. "Men could cook and wash and spin, and the women could do almost any kind of man's work. The girls could yoke up the cattle and go out and haul a load of wood, and sometimes when the girls were not in the field they would go and shoot a mess of squirrels and make a big pot-pie for their brothers' dinner. Where there were large families, the parents did but little, the boys and girls done nearly all."

"History shows us that while many women lived in the Victorian Age, they were not 'Victorian women'." (Carr) These women worked hard on the farms where they spent most of their lives. They didn't have the time or the leisure to sit around drinking afternoon tea, or to be concerned with whether or not a table's "limbs" were covered by a tablecloth. The submissive, virtuous, domestic woman was the ideal of nineteenth century American society – the ideal, not the reality.

CHAPTER FIVE
WOMEN IN THE NINETEENTH CENTURY

Rhoda Derry was born in tumultuous times. The nineteenth century was a confusing time to be a woman, with lots of mixed messages. The young country was experiencing its share of growing pains, and often, women were the ones caught in the middle.

At the beginning of the century, most production of goods was still a home-based industry. Work and home were the same place, whether a farmer was raising wheat or a housewife was making candles or clothes. But with the introduction of modern manufacturing methods, these two spheres began to diverge. Both men and women began to seek work outside the home. For women, this was largely unexplored territory.

One of the factors in this shift was the westward migration of the nineteenth century. As many men moved west to seek their fortunes, women moved into the jobs the men left behind. Children, too, were recruited. Women and children were used to doing the manual labor necessary to keep a farm and household running smoothly. When America shifted from an agrarian economy to a manufacturing economy, women and children formed the bulk of the new labor force.

WOMEN IN THE INDUSTRIAL REVOLUTION

In both Britain and America, it was textiles that led to the industrialization of the country. The success of the textile industry in New England was the bedrock on which America's dominance as an industrial nation was built.

There were three major reasons for women's ready acceptance into the grueling world of the cotton mills of New England. First, clothmaking was traditionally considered women's work. Before the Industrial Revolution, cloth was made at home. The very word "spinster" originated in the fact that it was the unmarried women in a household who got stuck with the tedious chores of the clothmaking process – spinning wool into yarn for weaving, retting flax into linen, and the other boring tasks of turning raw materials into cloth.

The second reason was the aforementioned migration of men – lots of them – to the west. Families moved, of course, but many men struck out for the frontier on their own, leaving jobs open to be filled by women. And the third reason stems from the second. Since women were not considered to be the traditional breadwinners, factory owners felt justified in hiring them for substandard or "supplemental" wages.

Crappy pay notwithstanding, women in New England flocked to the mills. The factories founded in Lowell, Massachusetts, in 1822 were staffed mostly by women. By 1831, women made up nearly forty thousand of the fifty-eight thousand workers in the cotton industry. They were an endless supply of cheap labor, and remained so from 1830 to 1860. The wages of a mill worker, between $3 and $3.50 per week, were far higher than anything farm daughters could earn in their home towns. Most mill owners didn't even have to advertise for workers – as women left the workforce, either to marry or to seek positions either in teaching or domestic service, their places on the line were filled by word of mouth. Factories reached far into the countryside to gather their work force. Cash wages, paid weekly, were a powerful draw, and companies built boardinghouses for the women they recruited. Living away from home provided social as well as financial independence.

Many women didn't stay long at the mills anyway. Most left after a few months, staying only long enough to earn enough for a trousseau or to set up a household. A study of one mill in 1836 showed that out of 233 female employees, only eighteen of them stayed for six years or longer. Many were glad, at least in the beginning, for the opportunity. Rather than stay in a large family, earning nothing and being considered a drain on the household's resources, women now had the opportunity to become self-supporting.

Those were the big draws for many young women. Some worked to earn their own living without having to depend on their families; some worked to help support their families. And some worked to save money for the households they would start when they got married. It wasn't poverty that pushed many young women into mill work, but rather a chance for economic independence that just wasn't possible while living and working at home.

The presence of women in the new factory workforce also spurred social reform. By the second quarter of the century, textile mills were horrible places to work. In 1845, a female factory worker testified about her job in a New Hampshire mill before a legislative committee. Hours in the summer were 5 am to 7 pm. Women, children, and a few men spent twelve to fourteen hours a day manufacturing cotton cloth. Wages for women were a paltry $20 to $25 per month. In 1847, protesters in New Hampshire won the right to work a ten-hour day.

The forced camaraderie of spending so much time working together forged a strong bond between female factory employees. They stood together to strike against unfair working conditions. Their backbone lent strength to social protest, too. Women reformers came to see parallels between black slavery and wage slavery, and protested them both. The women's rights conventions that had their birth in Seneca Falls, New York, in July 1848, led to a broad perspective on reform that came to include labor protest.

The experience of female mill workers demonstrates that the opening of factories to women not only brought women's work out of the home, but also encouraged women to participate in broader social reform.

WOMEN IN TEACHING

Before the nineteenth century, teachers were overwhelmingly male. But with the long, long reach of the Second Great Awakening and the idea of women being the center of the home, there was a shift toward thinking of women as teachers. It began with women being encouraged to guide their children at home, usually in a spiritual sense. But women parlayed this into permission to teach outside the home. Women were also seen as more virtuous, and able to set a better example for impressionable youth.

In 1845 Catherine Beecher wrote an elegant, widely-published article entitled "The Duty of American Women to Their Country", which stressed that the population was growing quickly – the mass of children needing a good education would soon outstrip the number of male teachers available to teach them. Therefore, it was up to women to take up the mantle of "teacher" and fill the breach. Teaching, she said, was a more rewarding way of earning a living than toiling in a factory, and more mentally stimulating than spending idle time in shopping, dressing for afternoon tea, and trading gossip.

Teaching, too, was an area in which women of the nineteenth century excelled. Historians estimate that in Massachusetts, for example, one out of every five women taught school at least once in her life by the middle of the century. By 1870, more than half of the two hundred thousand primary and secondary school teachers in America were female. Teaching, like factory work, gave women a taste of independence before they settled down and got married. It was less dangerous than working in a factory, and less monotonous than farm chores.

This isn't to say that teaching was a path to easy riches. Wages for female teachers were, at best, sixty percent of wages for male teachers. Wages were so low that many school districts followed the custom of "living in", where a teacher would board for a week or a month at a time with different families (usually the families of the school board), sharing their home and food. By the middle of the century, women dominated grammar school teaching, but they were slow to be hired in high schools and colleges, and completely excluded from any supervisory posts. It wasn't until the end of the century that women were allowed to serve on school boards and to take administrative positions.

Women teachers were also held to extremely high standards of social and moral behavior. They were not allowed to marry, at the cost of their jobs. A wife, after all, was supposed to stay home and run her household, not work outside the home. If married, a teacher should ideally be a widow, so that she could devote her full attention to the education of her pupils. Schoolrooms themselves – the one room affairs – were never to be used for dancing or games of chance, even in the off hours when students were not around. Teachers were forbidden to smoke, wear bright colors, hang out at the ice cream parlor in town, or wear skirts that came higher than two inches above the ankle.

THE RISE OF WOMEN'S MAGAZINES

Ironically, there was a group of women who made their careers out of the celebration of the home. Because "true women" needed advice and refinement, an entire industry of domesticity professionals developed in the nineteenth century. Nowhere was this more evident, or influential, than in the explosion of women's magazines.

In the years before the Civil War, magazines written especially for women flourished. These periodicals discussed nearly every subject under the sun (although they stayed strictly away from politics). Women could turn to magazines for advice on domestic economy, health and recreation, fashion, motherhood, and social reform, much as they do today. In fact, some of the magazines founded in the nineteenth century are still going strong – *McCall's*, *Ladies Home Journal*, and *Good Housekeeping* are still on magazine racks today.

By far the most influential of these was *Godey's Lady's Book*. With a run from 1830 to 1878, it was the most widely circulated magazine in the United States before the Civil War. It was glorified with the title "queen of monthlies".

And Sarah Josepha Hale was the queen of *Godey's Lady's Book*. She was the editor from 1837 to 1877, and the magazine grew remarkably in the forty years it was under her editorship. When she took the reins, circulation was at 10,000; two years later it had swelled to 40,000, and by 1860 it had topped 150,000. Hale used her powers as editor to further women's causes, as well as becoming the nineteenth century's leading arbiter of fashion and taste. She created the "Employment for Women" column in the magazine in 1852 to discuss women in the workforce.

Godey's Lady's Book was highly influential in matters of style. Queen Victoria is commonly credited with starting the tradition of wearing a white wedding dress, at her 1840 wedding to Prince Albert. She is also credited with introducing the Christmas tree to American households.

A woodcut illustration of the British royal family gathered around their Christmas tree was published by the *Illustrated London News* in 1848. It was republished in *Godey's Lady's Book* in the December 1850 issue, with a few Americanizing tweaks – namely, removing Victoria's crown and erasing Albert's mustache. This image was the first picture widely circulated in America of a Christmas tree with all the trimmings. *Godey's Lady's Book* set the tone for nostalgic Christmases for years to come, reprinting the image in 1860. By the 1870s, Christmas trees were a common part of American holiday celebrations.

Godey's Lady's Book was also key in creating another holiday – this one quintessentially American. The innovative Sarah Josepha Hale presented a series of eye-catching, mouth-watering articles, featuring descriptions of "typical" Thanksgiving food such as roast turkey, savory stuffing, and pumpkin pies. She even printed the recipes. At Hale's request, President Lincoln finally declared a national Day of Thanksgiving in 1863. But Hale had been banging her drum for thirty-six years by then.

The owner of the periodical, Louis Godey, insisted the magazine stay away from politics – undoubtedly a wise choice during the heated years of the Civil War. Hale, though, had a wealth of other subjects to explore. The pages of *Godey's Lady's Book* read like an AP English textbook, graced by such authors as Nathaniel Hawthorne, Harriet Beecher Stowe, Henry Wadsworth Longfellow, Ralph Waldo Emerson, Washington Irving, Oliver Wendell Holmes, and Edgar Allan Poe, whose "Cask of Amontillado" appeared in the magazine in 1846. The periodical was noted for its colored fashion plates, and even published needlework patterns and sheet music for piano.

Women's magazines, for the most part, focused on homemaking and encouraged their readers to do the same. Advertisers found out that the woman in a traditional, home-centered role was their best customer. She tended to buy the clothes, cosmetics, and household products the advertisers were hawking. She had interest in their wares, and even more importantly, the household budget to afford them. So, the companies with goods to sell tended to patronize magazines that focused on encouraging women to keep a tidy house and preside over it with elegance. These magazines went a long way towards elevating household management, defining the running of a household as a job requiring skill and intelligence. However, even as they helped women develop those domestic skills, they hindered women's journey towards exploration of trades outside the home.

MIXED MESSAGES

The mid-nineteenth century must have been a very difficult, confusing time to be a woman. On one hand, a woman had feminists like Elizabeth Cady Stanton, Lucretia Mott, and Amelia Bloomer fighting for women's rights. Women were allowed and even encouraged to work outside the home, albeit for long hours and dismal wages. However, those jobs were largely limited to menial labor in mills and garment factories, domestic jobs as maids, or teaching. Teachers, especially, were required to hold themselves to high standards of morality, dignity, and purity, to be a good example to the young students whose minds they were shaping. Teachers could not marry, under penalty of losing their job. Married women had one function – to bear children. And a pregnant schoolteacher would have thrown the Victorians into fits. If you're pregnant, you've obviously had sex. And what kind of example would *that* set?

Add the raging mid-nineteenth century debate over dress reform to these stresses, and women's lives got even more complicated. Cartoons and editorials ridiculed women's simple request to wear something *comfortable*, for heaven's sake. Amelia Bloomer, with her sensible Turkish trousers and loose tunic, was lambasted in the press, along with women who dared to shed their corsets and petticoats and follow her example. Men, of course, feared that the "loosening" of female dress codes would lead to immorality.

Meanwhile, as always, women of every class were overwhelmed with the demands of running a household, raising a family, and the stresses of childbearing and domesticity. We women today think it's difficult to be a "domestic goddess" – the folks in the nineteenth century took the phrase to a whole new level. It's no wonder that many women suffered physical and emotional breakdowns under the strain. Nervous disorders were so common as to be nearly epidemic for middle-class women by the late nineteenth century.

And all of this was far out of reach for the teenaged Rhoda Derry. She lived in a small town in a heavily agrarian part of the Illinois frontier. She never had the opportunity to work in a factory, the way her big-city sisters did. It's unlikely any family in Lima could have afforded to hire her as a domestic worker. She may have paged through an issue of Godey's Lady's Book, but she couldn't afford any of the cosmetics or fancy clothes advertised. And she didn't have a prayer of earning her own dowry.

Charles would just have to love her on her own merits.

PART TWO: THE COURTSHIP

CHAPTER SIX
YOUNG LOVE

Rhoda lies back on the blanket Charles has thoughtfully provided, and twines her fingers through his. The hay in the barn makes an adequate bed for their hasty, furtive meetings, but Rhoda longs for the comfort of her own marriage bed, the bed she will finally share with Charles as husband and wife.

"Have you asked them yet?" she whispers as Charles kisses the ticklish part of her neck, just under her ear.

Charles sits up, and Rhoda sighs inwardly. It is time, it really is time for him to approach his parents about the marriage. She has the sinking feeling that the longer Charles waits, the harder it will be for him to get their permission. Especially from Mrs. Phenix – Rhoda shudders. Nancy Phenix has the habit of wrinkling her nose whenever Rhoda sits at table with the family, as though she is trying to place the source of a faint but nasty smell.

"Are you ashamed of me?" Rhoda asks into the silence.

"No!" Charles yelps. "No, I love you, I want to be with you."

Rhoda sits up suddenly, pulling the dusty blankets around her bare shoulders. "Then why won't you marry me?" she spits.

Miserable, he plunges his hands through his hair, making it stand up at the crazy angles she finds so endearing. "I can't. Not until my parents give us their blessing."

Rhoda's heart sinks. It was the answer she has been expecting – and dreading. "Your mother will never give us her blessing. Never," she sobs, one hand fisted against her mouth.

She reaches for her blouse and shoves her arms into the sleeves. Her mind seethes as she tries to collect her racing, panicked thoughts. She can't lose Charles. She just can't. But his mother ... Mrs. Phenix hates her. She can feel it in every disapproving sniff, every dismissive glance.

"We'll run away together," Charles says suddenly. "That's what we'll do. We'll run away." He leans over, catches the back of Rhoda's head, and pulls her to *him for a deep, passionate kiss. She is smiling through her tears when she finally pulls away, the taste of him still on her lips, making her senses reel.*

But as she pins her hair up into the loose, untidy bun she favors, she worries.

In the eighteenth century, around ten percent of American brides came to the altar already pregnant with their first child. During the 1780s and 1790s, as many as one-third of the young women marrying in rural New England were also expecting. This was considered perfectly fine, as long as the couple then ended up marrying.

With the arrival of the nineteenth century, though, American attitudes toward morality underwent a significant change. Again looking at those same New England towns, by 1840 there were fewer than one in five premarital pregnancies. By 1860, the rate had plummeted to one in twenty.

This move toward stricter moral and sexual codes was a result of a change in attitude toward women. The first half of the nineteenth century saw the rise of the sentimental domestic ideal. American women were held up as examples of purity. The home was their domain.

Part of this was a result of the Second Great Awakening. The first quarter of the nineteenth century saw an evangelical revival that touched nearly every aspect of life. Faith was a critical concern to the female members of a family. As the goddesses of this new cult of domesticity, the caretakers of home and hearth, women felt themselves responsible for the spiritual welfare of their family, as well as its physical and emotional welfare. Young women in particular were drawn to participate in the Second Great Awakening. Ministers soon came to realize that their message was most effective when directed not at a family's patriarch, but at the women, the spiritual guardians of the household.

Evangelical revivals also gave women one of their few opportunities for autonomy. Giving themselves to religious devotion gave women the chance to take control, to state a preference.

On the frontier, church provided not only a social outlet, but also a means for charitable activity. Frontier communities often lacked voluntary associations like men's fraternal organizations or women's charity groups. Churches were often the best source of charity on the frontier.

Social consciousness flourished in the early decades of the nineteenth century, helped along by the Second Great Awakening. This was the beginning of the fight for equal rights for women. Even so, female moral crusaders were forced to soft-pedal their message of equality, just to get heard. They had to compromise their message in order not to alienate their male supporters.

These crusaders, women like Elizabeth Cady Stanton and Lucretia Mott, didn't argue against the way things were. They merely insisted that Christian principles be obeyed. They preached the sanctity of motherhood, the importance of purity for women, the delicacy of the fairer sex. They also insisted that a woman's place was in the home, at the center of the domestic sphere. And this is where these early moral reformers shot themselves in the foot. The more women threw themselves into public reform campaigns, the less effective was their rhetoric that women should remain isolated, reigning over their domestic kingdoms.

Even the rise of spiritualism affected American attitudes toward sex and marriage. Spiritualists believed that true love was the basis of marriage. Therefore, sexual intercourse as an expression of true love was completely natural and good. Sex wasn't purely carnal – love sanctified sexual intercourse and lifted it to the realm of heavenly passion.

Most religions, of course, taught that the soul was eternal. Spiritualism added the belief that the eternal soul was forever entwined with its ties on earth; thus the spiritualist vogue for contacting the dead. Spiritualism theorized that death was not an end, but a transition to a different phase of being. Mothers, devastated at the loss of a child, would remain that child's guardian in the life beyond this one.

But what about husbands and wives? Spiritualism taught that there was one person fated to be a spiritual mate through life and beyond, into eternity. But what if your spouse made you miserable? What if, after you got married, you met someone else, someone who completed you? What happened if you realized that your soul mate was someone other than your legally-bound partner?

Spiritualism was also, oddly enough, intimately connected with women's rights. Most mediums were young women, as women were seen as the more passive sex, more receptive to messages from the Other Side. And women's rights as an organized social movement began in Spiritualist homes. The table in Seneca Falls on which Elizabeth Cady Stanton and Lucretia Mott wrote the Declaration of Sentiments in 1848 was one used for rappings from beyond the veil.

In the years around 1850, social reformers and advocates for change introduced a new sexual theory that put sex front and center in relationships. State governments were revamping legal codes and replacing common law marriage.

Marriage became, in the eyes of the state, a lifelong contract unless ended by divorce.

Utopian communities also flourished in the first half of the nineteenth century, adding even more mixed messages about sexuality. The Shakers enjoyed a heyday during that time. They practiced celibacy and strictly segregated the sexes in both work and life.

At the other end of the spectrum, there was the Oneida colony in upstate New York, founded by John Humphrey Noyes. It still exists today; nowadays, they make silverware. But back in 1848, it was the scene of a spiritual adventure called "complex marriage", meaning that everyone in the colony was married to each other. Monogamy was soundly rejected. Childbearing decisions were handled by committee, who paired couples off just for the sake of procreation. Mothers cared for their children only for the first few years of life, at which time the entire community raised children.

Noyes had a reason for developing this system of "Male Continence and Complex Marriage". Within the span of six years, his wife had given birth to five children, four of whom were stillborn. Noyes' theories of cohabitation were intended to promote a more voluntary pattern of motherhood.

The freethinker Frances Wright rented a building in New York and named it the New York Hall of Science. It was her dream to have a hall of science in every city, to serve as a secular meeting place containing libraries, museums, and classrooms. Wright's lectures regularly packed the Hall's auditorium, with a seating capacity of more than 1,200.

The Hall was designed to be a social center for freethinkers and the working class. A free medical clinic for laborers was open every day. The Hall also housed a library and bookstore at the front of the building. The bookstore, defiantly open on Sundays, featured books by the rabble-rousing Thomas Paine and Percy Bysshe Shelley, a poet of questionable morality as far as polite society was concerned. These books were soon joined by a controversial work by the British author Richard Carlile. First printed in 1826, Carlile's *Every Woman's Book* was the first book published in Britain to give clear, unambiguous instructions on birth control.

Frances Wright also ran a newspaper, the *Free Enquirer*, along with fellow radical Robert Owen. In late October 1830, Owen announced to the paper's readers that he had written a book, and in early 1831 his book *Moral Physiology* was published. This was the first book written and produced in America that discussed contraception. By March 1831, the book had gone through two printings and was working on the third.

Contraception wasn't unknown in the nineteenth century. The educated classes, especially, were aware of the concept of family planning, or "voluntary motherhood". Wealthy families could afford more children; poor families needed more children to help around the house and help support the family when they were old enough to work. The middle class, though, realized the value of limiting family size. An educated couple who were financially comfortable wanted to keep it that way; by limiting the number of children, they could better live within their means.

The first half of the nineteenth century saw a drastic change in social consciousness. Women were placed on pedestals, becoming shining examples of domestic bliss and moral purity. Crusaders for women's rights saw this as a step forward, even as it trapped women in an amber of perfect homemaking. Contraception began to come out of the shadows. Utopian communities experimented with relationships in nearly every combination, from celibacy to complex marriage.

And all Rhoda and Charles wanted to do was get married.

We don't know how far Charles and Rhoda's relationship went. We do know that in 1852, when they had been courting for two years, Charles asked Rhoda to marry him.

The young lovers were both eighteen, which seems a bit young for marriage to us. And it was, even by the standards of the nineteenth century. By the 1860s, most Americans were in their early to mid-twenties when they wed. But Charles and Rhoda grew up on the frontier, not in one of the big cities of the East. They were well away from even the sophistication of Chicago or Springfield.

These two kids, both from small towns, knew their choices for a partner were limited. They were probably both thrilled they'd found someone compatible.

In his book *Pioneer Life in Illinois*, F.M. Perryman describes frontier courtship. Perryman was born on the Illinois frontier in 1836, just two years after Charles and Rhoda, so their experience was likely similar to the memories Perryman set down in his book.

Perryman started his essay "No Divorce" by describing planting methods. The young men and women of the neighborhood would gather to plant corn in the spring. It was a cooperative effort; some would go along dropping seed, with others following behind to cover it.

"Sometimes a young man and young woman would meet in the field and stop and talk and sometimes make a bargain to get married ... and when they made an engagement, that engagement was made to stay. The divorce court got no work there; and when they got married, all the people for miles around would be there, and all would contribute something to make up a big dinner of the best that the country afforded. The men would get together and cut logs and build them a house and most every family for miles around would give them a quilt or blanket, or pillow, and soon they were pretty well fixed."

This was the blissful future Charles and Rhoda could have looked forward to – all their neighbors gathering for a celebration, and giving gifts to make sure the young couple was well set up for their new life together.

Unfortunately, there was someone who was dead set against the marriage. Nancy Phenix, Charles' mother, was furious that her son was even considering marrying one of the dirt-poor Derrys.

Nancy Phenix was from a different generation. In the past, parents often chose their children's spouses with an eye toward increasing the family's wealth or land holdings. But by the middle of the nineteenth century, most young people, and even many parents, believed men and women should marry for love. It was becoming perfectly acceptable to choose a partner based on mutual attraction, even romance.

This romantic ideal was reinforced by poetry and sentimental stories in women's magazines, like the *Ladies' Repository* and *Godey's Lady's Book*. These magazines fed the dreamy fantasies of many young women, describing long engagements, and encouraging prospective brides to collect impressive trousseaus. (The phrase "follow the money" is particularly apt here. Many of these publications were fashion magazines, which ran articles aimed at getting women to spend their disposable income on clothes.)

As the youngest child of a poor frontier family, with no income of her own, Rhoda would not have had the opportunity to indulge in such frivolities. But that doesn't mean she didn't daydream about being married to Charles, the love of her life. Teenage love is a tender, wondrous, volatile, explosive thing. The passion of a teenage girl burns hot and bright like newsprint. It flames up with an all-consuming fire. A teenage girl is a creature of powerful longings, of fierce adoration freely, unthinkingly given.

Imagine the young lovers, desperate to be together, but knowing one parent would never give her blessing to the union.

CHAPTER SEVEN
THE CONFRONTATION

Nancy Phenix scowls and drops the curtain over the kitchen window. That Derry girl is coming up the road from the barn – again! As if she thought Nancy didn't know she was stepping out with Charles. Nancy sniffs and turns away.

"That Derry girl's here again," she says.

Frederick grunts and turns the page of his newspaper.

"I don't like it, Frederick. I think Charles might be getting serious about her."

Frederick lowers the paper and gives his wife a mild look. "And?"

"And I won't have it!" Nancy bursts out. "You know her family is dirt poor! I'm not having my son take on the responsibility of a bunch of freeloading inlaws!"

Frederick shakes his head and goes back to reading his paper.

"Hmpf! Some confidante you are. Well, never mind. I'll just take care of this myself." She unties her apron, tosses it on the kitchen table, and heads for the door. She stops, her hand on the doorknob, and looks back at her husband.

"You'll thank me for this later, you know."

As Nancy strides out to meet Rhoda, she sees Charles following behind the girl like a love-struck bull calf. She snorts. They were coming from the barn – how stupid did they think she was? Did they honestly think she didn't know what they got up to in there? She sets her jaw. It was just as well Charles is here too, tagging along behind his lady love. No use prolonging the inevitable. Nancy is fully prepared to put an end to this nonsense. A cruel smile plays on her face.

She knows exactly how to do it, too.

Nancy steps in front of the Derry girl, blocking her path. The girl has been walking with her head down, but Nancy claims her attention. Charles, following several steps behind her, hurries to catch up.

"Mother! What are you –"

"Be quiet, Charles. You don't know what you're doing. This girl is evil – her whole family is rotten to the core. And –" she draws herself up with a glare of righteous indignation, "—her grandmother was a witch. Blood will out, in people just as much as in horses. You ought to know that."

"Mother, no!" Charles yelps. "That can't be true. Rhoda is innocent of such things." He takes Rhoda's hand and faces his mother, defiance written in his young face.

"We've had enough of your rumors and lies. That's all you're willing to believe. Well, we've had enough. I'm going to take Rhoda, and we're going to run away together."

Nancy's eyes narrow in fury. "This you will not do, Charles! I forbid it. I forbid it and I will put a stop to this foolishness once and for all!"

Nancy draws herself up to her full height and raises her hands to the sky. She steals a quick glance at the Derry girl, and is pleased to see a look of sick recognition on her face. Nancy lets a tone of menace flow through her words.

"I forbid you and Charles to marry. If you continue to see my son, I will put a curse on you," she intones.

"Please," Rhoda bursts out, "please, Mrs. Phenix, I love Charles, we want to be together and my father has given us his blessing. Please do not do this. I can't bear to be without him!"

Nancy allows herself a moment of satisfaction. She relishes the note of terrified panic in the girl's voice. This will teach the little chit. She lowers her arms, then points at Rhoda.

"I have warned you. You refused to listen. Instead, you and Charles continue to defy me. Now, a curse is upon you. You will never spawn any evil from my son's loins. Now go – I am finished with you." She drops her arm and turns away from Rhoda, hiding a smile. She hears the thud of high-button shoes on the hard-packed earth of the road as the girl flees.

"Mother, what did you do?" Her son's voice is rough with anguish. Nancy straightens her shoulders, then turns to face Charles. It is hard, but sometimes a mother has to do what needs to be done to protect her children.

"You're well rid of her," she says. Her voice softens as she takes in the tears welling in Charles' eyes. "You'll thank me for this later."

The big muscles in Rhoda's legs burn as she pounds down the road. Charles' house is a pleasant afternoon's stroll from hers, not far at all, and if she runs she can get home fast fast fast but she doesn't want to get home she doesn't want to yes she does she wants to get home and throw herself on her bed and cry her eyes out and kick and scream and cry because she is dying dying inside because she is never going to see her Charles again, ever, he probably hates her now that she is cursed, she is cursed and she is going to die anyway so what does it matter?

A stitch in her side slides a butter knife between her ribs so she slows to a trot, her chest still heaving. Her mind scrabbles like a panicked mouse running the closed track of her skull, seeking a way out of this misery, but trapped, trapped, trapped with the agony that will never go away.

Her hair has come loose from its bun and is hanging in lank, sweaty strands in her face. She is trotting past the old Youngquist place now, only three houses to go until she can run upstairs to her room and curl up in a ball and never never wake up. She doesn't want to look at it, it is abandoned and spooky and there are weeds growing up around the windows. "Don't look, Rhoda, don't look, Rhoda, don't look," she pants under her breath.

But she does look, she does, and there he is, grinning out of the broken window at her, the glass slicing his black face in half, grinning with too many teeth and then he is crawling out of the window down the gray wall, all teeth and spindly legs and long fingers with too many joints and claws, oh god it's Old Scratch just like in Granny Moll's stories and he is coming for her he is coming for little Rhody he is going to come and eat her up and crunch her bones and finally yes she is home and she pounds up the stairs and she is falling falling falling until she lands in softness, she is safe in her bed for now but she won't ever really be safe ever again, not without Charles. She yanks the blankets up under her chin and she cries and she doesn't come out again for a very long time.

PART THREE: THE DECLINE

CHAPTER EIGHT
MOLL DERRY

What happened to Rhoda? What makes a young, healthy mind snap so completely?

In order to understand Rhoda's first, tragic break with reality, we need to look farther back in her history than her confrontation with Nancy Phenix. We need to look two generations back, to Rhoda's grandmother, Mollie Derry. Rhoda's story is fascinating and tragic. And it reaches out beyond her lifetime – in both directions. Rhoda's story starts even before her birth.

It starts with the birth of our nation.

The British officer strolls out of the open gate of the stockade. He'll be leading a skirmishing party in less than an hour, and it will be good to stretch his legs before then.

He spares a glance at the tree line, a hundred and fifty yards away. Nothing's moving over there. He turns back to the stockade.

A crack echoes across the valley. The officer grunts and falls to his knees, a crimson stain blooming on the cardinal red of his uniform. A moment later he pitches forward and lies still.

In the tree line, two sharpshooters nod with satisfaction. One of them, taller than the second, looks around quickly. Seeing no one, he stoops and brushes a quick, congratulatory kiss on the shorter one's cheek.

"Well done, Mollie," he mutters, and the slightly built sharpshooter blushes with pleasure at the compliment. Because one of Morgan's Riflemen ... is a riflewoman.

Molly Pitcher. Sybil Ludington. Betsy Ross. There were many women who were as passionately patriotic as the Founding Fathers were. All of them had adventures in the tumultuous days of the American Revolution. Some of them even became folk heroines, their stories passed down in grade school textbooks. But there is one Revolutionary War heroine whose story is a bit more complicated than can be told in a children's picture book.

Valentine Derry, also known as Felty, and Mary Derry, called Moll, were married and living in Germany at the time of the American Revolution. Moll was born anywhere between 1760 and 1768. An earlier birthdate makes more sense; if she was born in 1760, she'd have been sixteen years old in 1776, when the war broke out.

What did a war thousands of miles away in the New World have to do with the Derrys? Plenty. Great Britain conscripted soldiers for the war from many of the German states, according to the treaties Prussia had signed with Britain. The state of Hesse-Kassel contributed the most men to the British cause, so Americans started calling the German soldiers "Hessians". All told, 30,000 Germans fought for Britain during the Revolutionary War.

So Valentine was conscripted and sent to the colonies to fight. Mollie, a young bride, had no intention of being left behind in Germany. She disguised herself as a man to travel with Valentine.

When the two arrived in Virginia, Mollie continued her subterfuge. Valentine Derry was also, as things turned out, one of 4,888 German troops who deserted the British. Valentine defected to fight for the Americans. And Mollie went with him, to fight at his side.

Mollie, still in disguise as a man, and Valentine both joined Morgan's Riflemen. At the time, Daniel Morgan was living in Charles Town, Virginia (now West Virginia), just a stone's throw across the line into Loudon County, Virginia. He commanded the Eleventh Virginia Regiment.

Members of Morgan's Riflemen had to pass a test of certain sharpshooter skills. They did not wear uniforms, but rather hunting clothing – leggings and moccasins – with a feather worn in the cap. They were deadly with the flintlock rifle, and the group was instrumental in winning several battles during the war.

A passage in the *Military Journal of the Revolution*, written in August 1775, describes the battalion: "These men are remarkable for the accuracy of their aim; striking a mark with great certainty at two hundred yards' distance. At a review, a company of them, while on a quick advance, fired their balls into objects of seven inches diameter, at a distance of two hundred and fifty yards." A sharpshooter using a rifle could make a shot more than twice as long a distance as an infantryman using a musket.

Ancestry.com puts the Derrys' arrival in America sometime in November 1783. This may be a bit late, as the Revolutionary War ended in September of that year. Nonetheless, Derry family lore has Mollie fighting alongside Valentine during the war. This is echoed in a newspaper article from the *Mountain Democrat*. The article was published in 1879, thirty-six years after Mollie's death in 1843.

The article described Valentine's prowess as a hunter. It was "Old Moll" who became known as a witch, but Valentine had quite the reputation as a hunter with preternatural powers.

"It was thought by 〚many〛 persons that he was a wizard, and could charm the deer. He sometimes used a certain ingredient that he rubbed on his moccasins and leggings. He would then make a circuit where deer were plenty, and take his position some twenty-five or thirty steps at either side. In a short time he would see a buck coming on a slow trot. When at a proper range he would bleat, the deer would stop, and he was always sure of his meat. If he wanted another one he never had to wait long. He once tracked an old she bear, that had cubs, in the rocks. After some deliberation he concluded to crawl in and shoot her in the den. She met him half way at a narrow passage. He lying down, and she coming out, fastened on him and commenced eating her way out; but before she had done any more damage than tearing the seat out of his leather breeches, he got his hunting knife out of his scabbard that was at 〚his〛 side, and plunged it into her, behind the fore shoulder, and she lay on him a lifeless bear."

After the war, the Derrys moved from the Loudon County, Virginia, over the Allegheny Mountains, to Fayette County, Pennsylvania. It was here that they started a family. The "Fortune Teller of the Revolution" was also a mother. Between 1793 and 1811, Valentine and Mollie had seven children – Bazil (1793), Jacob (1795), Barbara (1798), Philip (around 1800), Jerimiah (1802), Rhoda (1804), and Mary (1811).

Moll's oldest son, Bazil Derry, took after both of his parents. He became known, in his own right, as "a great hunter with excellent sharpshooter skills", and wore handmade moccasins he had sewn himself.

It was while living in Fayette County that Moll Derry began her practice as a healer – and a hexer. The gun-toting, varmint-shooting wife of Valentine Derry, who crossed an ocean and dressed as a man to fight at her husband's side, added another facet to her already complicated personality. She became a practitioner of Pennsylvania Dutch hex magic.

WITCHCRAFT AND HEX MAGIC

In the years before modern medicine, the practice of folk magic gave its practitioners a sense of control in an uncertain and savage world. This very personal style of magical work was a mélange of techniques – fortunetelling, spells for protection of farm animals and property, and removal of curses and hexes. The use of healing herbs was also a big part of folk magic. Herbal medicine was the practical foundation of the natural laws on which folk magic was built.

Pennsylvania, especially the southwestern part of the state, was fertile soil for the development of hex magic. A lot of Quakers settled in the state. Their general tolerance of many different religious beliefs attracted numerous German immigrants to the area. Some of these immigrants were members of religious groups much more obscure than the Quakers.

These uprooted Germans also tended to a strong belief in witchcraft and the supernatural. Look at the rich tapestry of folk tales woven by the Brothers Grimm. Imagine the dark, haunted forests of old Germany, inhabited by hungry wolves, talking bears, and witches eager to lure unsuspecting children to their doom with enticing cabins built of gingerbread. Then imagine those wild forests transplanted across the Atlantic to America. Here, the forests reached not only to the border of France, Poland, or Austria, but for thousands of miles to the west, as far as one's imagination could reach, and beyond.

The practice of Pennsylvania Dutch hex magic, also known as powwowing, can be divided into two paths: braucherei, which is healing, blessing, and charms for good luck and prosperity, and hexerai, which is casting curses. As a powerful magic worker, Moll would have needed to be an expert in both lifting and casting curses. This would have made her both respected and feared. Moll Derry was no one to be trifled with.

The people who could live in harmony with this supernatural landscape were regarded with healthy respect, tinged with a fair amount of fear. They were considered to have supernatural abilities, but they weren't persecuted as in Salem a hundred and twenty years previously. People on the frontier were too busy carving a living from the Pennsylvania forest to worry about accusing a neighbor of souring the milk. The settlers of southwestern Pennsylvania were a more pragmatic bunch than the paranoid Puritans of Massachusetts, who jumped at every witch-shaped shadow. Besides, these folks had real powers, powers they used for good as well as ill. On the frontier, it was taken as read that if you crossed a powwower, he or she would hex you. The trick was to stay on their good side.

According to Pennsylvania Dutch tradition, the difference, put simply, between the witch and the powwower is that the witch's power comes from the devil, and the powwower's abilities come from God. The powwower gives God the credit for his or her success, while the witch simply takes the credit and leaves God out of the picture. Witches were feared and excluded from the community. Powwowers were respected members of the community, and considered to be almost holy due to their healing partnership with God.

There is a Christian element to the practice of powwow, as well as a magical element. This blend of ritual blessing and use of blessed objects within a population that is predominantly Protestant seems to suggest that hex magic may have its roots in Roman Catholic practice that moved underground after the Reformation. The Protestant Reformation not only severed itself from the Pope and from Catholic hierarchy, it also rejected the Catholic use of symbols to represent religious concepts.

The Protestant church authorities also moved away from the concept of religious healing. No more would they place their faith in the curative powers of a relic, or of holy water. That was left to the Catholics. Folk healing was driven underground, to become the province of lay practitioners. It's interesting that the most vocal opponents of powwowing, in modern times, belong to radical Protestant groups – the Mennonites and Old Order Amish. There are members of these groups that still practice folk magic, but they keep it on the down low.

The relationship between physician and folk magic practitioner was much closer in the eighteenth and nineteenth centuries, when Moll Derry was casting her spells, than it is today. Today, we want to separate "real medicine" from superstition. But two hundred years ago, physicians grew their own herbs and prepared remedies from them, much like powwowers did. Neither powwowers nor most rural physicians charged for their diagnostic or healing services, only for the materials used. Most physicians didn't have formal medical training anyway. Up until the middle of the twentieth century, physicians would refer patients to powwowers for treatment. Likewise, powwowers would bring their incantations and paraphernalia into hospitals to perform hex magic over patients.

Pennsylvania hex magic has survived to the present day. The philosophical descendants of Moll Derry are alive and well and practicing their magic in the hills and hollers of rural Pennsylvania.

Many powwow cures are written down in books such as *The Long Lost Friend*, a book by John George Hohman. First published in 1820, this is a collection of home remedies, herbal cures, and folk healing, along with more esoteric material such as spells and charms.

Today, every practitioner has his or her own way of training the next generation. Training can take anywhere between a few minutes to a year. With a more structured approach, the apprentice has to be able to repeat back every lesson learned in every previous training session. Incantations that have to be memorized are mostly in English, but some are in German or in Pennsylvania Dutch. This method of cumulative memorization ensures that when the apprentice strikes out on their own, they can perform the complicated hand movements and recite the spells without having to stop in the middle of the procedure to consult a book. This is meant to bolster the patient's confidence in the powwower.

Most powwow healing is performed very near the patient, with the healer's hands hovering close to the patient, almost but not quite touching. It's much like reiki healing in its use of energy work. Many procedures used in healing rituals are repeated three times, in a nod to the Holy Trinity of Christian theology. The incantations also include the "three holiest names": Father, Son, and Holy Ghost. Perhaps out of reverence for the intercession of such powerful beings, the incantations in a powwow are mumbled so low that only the healer can understand them. The patient, even though she is right there being worked on and prayed over, can't understand the magical summonings. To the patient, it must remain a mystery.

THE WHITE ROCKS

Moll Derry became widely known throughout southwestern Pennsylvania as a healer, working with roots and herbs. She gained great renown as a powwower, able to cast spells for harm as well as for healing. She was also said to have owned an Erd Spiegel ("earth mirror"), a sort of crystal ball by which she could foretell the future.

Moll made her reputation partly as a teller of fortunes. It was said she could find any item that was lost, "whether horse or cow, pocket-book, money, jewels, silver spoons, or any other thing of real or imaginary value". Many stories were told about Moll's ability, not only to find lost items, but also, if the item had been stolen, to give a description of the thief.

Moll's preferred method of divination was through the use of coffee grounds. Anyone who came to Moll's cabin to have their fortune told had to bring two things: money for the fee, and coffee. Moll brewed the coffee very strong, making sure to leave plenty of grounds. Moll would encourage the guest to have a leisurely drink.

"The cup being placed in the left hand of the seeker, bottom upwards, and the subject required to turn the cup three times, being careful to turn the cup toward the seeker, Mollie would then take the cup, and by the grounds that adhered to the sides and bottom, read off the seeker's fortune. It was thought by many that Mollie had intimate dealings with the devil. As far as known, she harmed no one, and if she got her money and coffee, she was always contented." (From the 1879 *Mountain Democrat* article.)

As Moll's reputation grew, so did the stories that swirled around Fayette County. Old Moll was described variously as a large woman, or as being so petite she slept in a cradle. She was said to "ride great distances on a broomstick", and she could command rattlesnakes to guard her and to watch over her cabin while she was away. Sometimes she was called Moll Derry, sometimes Moll Wampler. There are two reasons commonly given for this alias. One is that Moll herself used a fake name, to disguise her occult activities. Another possibility is that since many of the stories about Moll began to circulate while she was still very much alive, the storytellers used the name Moll Wampler to throw Moll Derry off their scent. Fearing they would anger her if they used her real name, they made up an alias for her. No one wanted to be on Moll Derry's bad side.

The legends are clear on this point. Moll Derry was not a woman to be crossed. According to the stories, Moll was not above a few traditionally witchy tantrums. If neighbors angered her, she supposedly made their cows sick, or stopped their bread from rising.

And Moll was apparently not always contented with her coffee. She could be fearsome when crossed. For many years, tales were told about Moll's power to curse. Many of these tales survive in the supernatural folklore of the area, where Moll is known even today as a witch.

In the mid-1790s, Moll ran into three men who taunted her about her abilities. Moll was furious, and told the men that all three of them would hang. One of the men, whose last name was either McFall or Butler, killed a man in a drunken fight in 1795. He was quickly arrested, convicted of the murder, and hanged. He was, supposedly, the first man to be executed in Fayette County by hanging.

The next of the three men to hang was named Dougherty. After murdering a man in Fayette County, he fled to Ohio. He killed again – but this time, he got caught. He confessed to both murders, was convicted, and was hanged in 1800.

The third man, whose name may have been Flanigan, learned what had happened to his two companions. Remembering Moll Derry's curse, he realized what his eventual fate would be. He committed suicide ... by hanging himself.

Wilbur R. Landman supplied some of these "Old Moll" stories to Joan Brown Derry, one of the family's historians. Landman's grandparents knew Moll Derry personally. She ran a "granny store" where Landman's grandparents bought sundries. Landman's great-grandmother Cunningham often told stories about "Old Moll". "She was a real witch," Cunningham swore.

One of her talents was detecting the guilty. Wilbur Landman passed along an incident that happened in the spring of 1818 or 1819. A peddler was passing through Smithfield and stopped at a tavern for some refreshment. While he was there, he ran into an acquaintance of his named John Updyke. The peddler was actually planning to stop in and see Moll Derry to have his fortune told. Updyke helpfully promised to take the man to Old Moll's cabin. He led the peddler to his own cabin instead. There, he and his friend Ned Cassidy robbed the man and killed him.

Updyke and Cassidy were members of a gang from McClellandtown that operated around Smithfield. Their tactics were to rob Shaker farmers coming home from the market, relieving them of the money they had made selling their goods. The Shakers and Mennonites of the area were easy prey, because they didn't carry guns. The gang would accost the farmers, rob them, kill them, and dump their bodies in the millpond at Rubles Mill. The traveling peddler met the same awful fate.

Eventually, though, it seems that Cassidy had an attack of conscience. He went to see Moll on his own, seeking a potion that would help him sleep. When he came to her cabin, Moll supposedly said, "Why are you coming to me when your hands are still wet from your dirty work at the millpond?" Cassidy was thrown badly by this accusation. He scurried off and escaped Moll's piercing gaze.

Updyke was not nearly so lucky. At that time, Old Moll had an apprentice named Hannah Clarke, who lived just up the road from Updyke. One day, a prominent citizen, who also knew Updyke, stopped in to pay Hannah a visit. He noticed a drawing on the back of the door, a sketch that resembled Updyke. There was a nail tapped into the head of the figure, with most of the nail still protruding from the door. Seeing the man looking at the drawing, Hannah explained that if she drove the nail all the way into the drawing, Updyke would die. So, she was tapping it in a little at a time, so he would suffer for his crimes.

The man's next stop was to visit Updyke. Oddly enough, Updyke complained of a headache – sort of a piercing pain. Updyke lingered for several weeks, as the pain in his head grew worse and worse. Soon he could no longer get out of bed. As he lay dying, he confessed to the murder of the peddler.

Not long after that, Hannah Clarke drove the nail all the way into the door.

Moll Derry made her way into fiction as well. A writer named A. F. Hill wove a story, based on true events, titled *The White Rocks*. It's the tragic story of Polly Williams, who in 1810 was killed by the man she had planned to marry. Polly was a beautiful young girl from a poor family that lived in New Salem. Polly took a job as a servant in the household of Jacob Moss. One of Moss' neighbors, Philip Rogers, was attracted to the pretty servant girl. In 1808, the rest of Polly's family moved west, but Polly stayed behind with Philip, hoping they would soon be married. But Philip kept postponing the wedding.

One day, while out for a walk near the White Rocks, Polly encountered Moll Derry. Moll offered to tell Polly's fortune, but reeled back in horror when she saw only blood and death. Moll warned Polly that Philip would end up hurling her off a ledge onto the rocks below.

This shook Polly enough that she confided in Mrs. Moss, saying she feared Philip would hurt her. Mrs. Moss tried to talk Polly into calling off the engagement, but inexplicably, Polly refused.

Late in the summer of 1810, Philip told Polly that he had arranged for a minister to marry them at the White Rocks. Polly was ecstatic, and rushed to put on her best dress and follow Philip into the woods. But it was all a ruse.

The next day, Polly Williams' body was found in the hollow below the White Rocks. The doctor's examination showed she had been struck on the head with a rock, then her body had been thrown from the cliff. Philip Rogers was charged with Polly's murder, but he hired talented lawyers and was acquitted. Polly was buried in the Little White Rock Cemetery, where people still visit her grave today. Her ghost is said to wander the ledges of the White Rocks, waiting for the man who would never marry her.

Such was Moll Derry's legend, she even showed up in stories that happened well after her death. In *The Lost Children of the Alleghenies* – again, a fictionalized account of true events that happened in 1856 – Moll Wampler uses her Erd Spiegel to try to find the two lost Cox brothers in Bedford County. She tells of seeing the children on the ground, either dead or sleeping. When the boys are found dead, an angry mob kills her out of frustration. (In reality, the boys, who had frozen to death, were discovered by a man who had a dream about their location.) While "Moll Wampler" took the fall in this story, Moll Derry died in 1843, before the boys were even born.

MOLLIE AND HER FAMILY

But before she was the fearsome "Old Moll", Mollie Derry was first and foremost a mother. She and Valentine had seven children, and those children would certainly have known about their mother's powwowing activities. Jacob, who would become Rhoda's father, was born in 1795 – about the time Moll had her run-in with the three men who later hanged after she pronounced her curse. Jacob married Rachel Bright in 1815, just a few years before the incident at the millpond, and Hannah Clarke's occult execution of John Updyke.

By 1822, Jacob and Rachel were well on their way to starting their own brood. Three of their children – Philip (1817), Basil (1820), and Carlisle (1822) – were born while Jacob and Rachel were living in Fayette County, Pennsylvania, presumably near Mollie. By 1824, though, Jacob had moved the family west to Indiana. Jacob and Rachel would have six more children during their years in Indiana: Margaret (1824), Mary Jane (1827), Jerimiah (1829), James McCann (1831), Barbara (1832), and finally Rhoda, the last to be born, in 1834.

The children were growing up quickly. Philip, the oldest son, moved to Illinois and married Cynthia Pribble. Basil married his first wife, Sarah "Sallie" Slater, in Indiana in 1841. Then they, too, moved west to Illinois. Mary Jane Derry married Anderson Slater, Sarah's older brother. Carlisle stayed in Indiana for a while, then married and moved to Missouri.

Sometime in 1843, after moving several times to different counties in Indiana, Jacob decided to join his two oldest sons in Illinois. He moved the family again, this time to Lima, in western Illinois just outside Quincy in Adams County.

The family's relationship with Mollie is puzzling. Doc Derry writes, "Certainly the pagan practices of Old Moll were well known to her children. My second great-grandparents, Jacob and wife, Rachel, surely understood and may have even practiced Mollie's witchery. Conceivably, Rachel herself was an apprentice of Old Moll's. Jacob and Rachel were, after all, living with or near Mollie after they were married for seven or eight years before moving on to Indiana." It's not out of line, either, to imagine Jacob being Moll's apprentice. In the powwowing tradition, practitioners can be either male or female. Sometimes, female practitioners will only take male apprentices, and vice versa.

But other historians claim it was Rachel who convinced Jacob to move away from Moll's influence. According to this theory, Rachel wanted nothing to do with "Old Moll". Rachel's antipathy could have instilled a deep fear of witches in Rhoda – a fear that Nancy Phenix later played upon, with disastrous results.

Mollie Derry passed away sometime before June 17, 1843. That's when Jacob Dawson, one of the witnesses to her will, testified before the Registrar for the probate that the will was in order. Jacob Derry was the other witness, but by 1843, he had moved to Illinois.

Mollie left everything she had to give – her house and lot in George Township in Fayette County – to her grandson, Andrew Derry. Andrew was the son of Mollie's youngest daughter, Mary (who was named executrix of the will). The will was written up, signed, and sealed on May 15, 1843, just about a month before it had to be proven in court. So sometime during that month, Mollie passed.

Mollie Derry probably never met her young granddaughter Rhoda. Rhoda was nine years old, and had just moved with her family to Illinois, when Mollie died. Before that, the family was living in Indiana, where Rhoda was born. With travel conditions on the frontier in the first half of the nineteenth century being somewhat dodgy, it's likely that the news of Rhoda's birth, along with the births of five of her older brothers and sisters, was relayed to Mollie by mail or via another message rather than in person.

With "Old Moll" having such an outsized personality, we can be sure that little Rhoda heard plenty of stories about her grandmother as she was growing up. Rhoda's three oldest brothers, Philip, Basil, and Carlisle, would have been cuddled on Mollie's lap as babies. Jacob and Rachel spent the first seven or eight years of their marriage living close to Mollie, so Philip and Basil surely would have had memories of their grandmother. (Carlisle, maybe not so much, as he was only two years old when the family moved to Indiana.) As older brothers, they probably delighted in scaring the stuffing out of their younger siblings with "Old Moll" spook tales.

It's possible, too, that Jacob and Rachel had "Old Moll" stories of their own, that they passed down to their nine children. We don't know the substance of these family legends. We do know, though, that Rhoda was deeply terrified of witchcraft. Maybe this bone-deep terror was instilled in her through repeated tellings of Old Moll's exploits.

And what would Old Moll herself have thought of her young granddaughter's affliction? The wise old woman, steeped as she was in both the light and dark side of folk magic, would most likely have clucked her tongue in sympathy, and pronounced a diagnosis of black witchcraft, a serious hex, or even demonic possession.

One wonders what cure Old Moll would have prescribed for her beloved granddaughter, and what retribution she would have called down upon Nancy Phenix for the trouble she had caused.

One also wonders if it would have worked.

CHAPTER NINE
WITCHES

Rhoda was not getting any better.

When Nancy Phenix pronounced her "curse" on Rhoda, she was only trying to stop Rhoda's marriage to Charles. She didn't mean to destroy Rhoda's life, or even cause her any lasting harm. But her carefully-chosen words caused Rhoda incalculable damage.

Nancy Phenix couldn't fail to see how Rhoda was suffering. In a small town like Lima or Ursa, news of a young woman's terrifying fits would have traveled at the speed of a prairie wildfire. Nancy must have realized fairly early on that the ruse had gone too far. Perhaps she felt guilty for making Rhoda believe so thoroughly that a curse had shattered her life.

Nancy even sought out one of Rhoda's brothers, trying to make amends. She stopped one of the brothers, possibly Jerimiah, on the road. She asked to be taken to see Rhoda, saying that she would release Rhoda from the "spell". Maybe she still wanted to prove her power over Rhoda; maybe she just used words that she felt Rhoda could understand. But whatever led Nancy to seek Rhoda out, it was far too late for the young woman.

A scream splits the air.

"Mama mama mama!" In the extremity of her terror, Rhoda is reduced to shrieking like a toddler. "The witches, Mama! They're coming, the witches are here, they're all around me!"

A crack echoes in the cabin, and a splinter of wood explodes from the corner of the ceiling. Five more shots follow – Rachel Derry is firing her pistol into the air to scare away the invisible witches. Rhoda crouches under the heavy wooden table, her hands over her ears, shivering in terror. The witches are imaginary, but to her, they are horrifyingly real.

The pistol is empty. Rachel drops it into the wide pocket of her apron and kneels to coax Rhoda from her hiding place. Rachel grabs for her daughter and holds her close as Rhoda clings to her, sobbing with mingled fear and relief. Rachel strokes her daughter's head, her fingers working their way through Rhoda's thick dark hair.

Was this a regular occurrence? We don't know for sure. It happened often enough to become entrenched in Derry family history. Did Rachel shoot at imaginary witches in response to an attempted visit from Nancy Phenix? Was this the best way to scare away the woman who'd cause her youngest daughter so much pain? Was Rachel perhaps letting off some of her own stress? Nancy Phenix was definitely not welcome in the Derry home. Did Rachel fire her pistol in the air to make that point abundantly clear?

Here's another interesting question: where was Charles Phenix during all of this? Where was he in the weeks and months after Rhoda's break with consensual reality? Nancy was undoubtedly keeping him away from Rhoda. But did he take it quietly? Or did he fight for the girl he loved?

Again, this is something we will never know for sure. But we do know this: Charles *loved* Rhoda. He loved her enough to ask her to marry him. It's difficult to imagine that kind of commitment could just disappear overnight. Perhaps he got scared away by Rhoda's break with reality. It's possible. When the "spell" that his mother cast on Rhoda seemed to have horrifyingly real results, Charles must have been stunned at this drastic change in the girl he loved.

We don't know what kind of relationship the Derrys had with the Phenixes. But we can make some educated guesses. Charles was a bright kid, self-possessed, intelligent – a great prospect for Rhoda. As the youngest child, she was likely the last to think about getting married, and her family was probably thrilled that the older son of the well-to-do Phenixes was interested in her.

Charles was a middle child, but the oldest son, which probably gave him confidence. He was responsible enough to act as a witness in an attempted murder case three years before he met Rhoda, when he was only thirteen.

Rhoda, in comparison, was the youngest of nine children. She was undoubtedly thrilled at the undivided attention Charles gave her.

Charles and Rhoda were each other's first love. Charles was confident enough in his feelings for Rhoda, and confident enough that she loved him back, that he proposed to her when they were both eighteen. That was a young age to be considering marriage at that time – most young men of the mid-nineteenth century didn't marry until later. The average age at marriage in 1850 was twenty-six for men, and twenty-three for women. Either Charles was besotted, or he was very secure in the relationship.

Charles proposed to Rhoda, and she accepted – which means both of them had most likely thought about the joining of their two families. Lima and Ursa were close enough that once Charles and Rhoda started courting, the families would have met. And Nancy knew enough about Rhoda's background to know that invoking witchcraft would have been an extremely effective way to get her attention.

Nancy Phenix was so dead set against this marriage that she was willing to pretend to cast a curse on Rhoda, even at the risk of being accused of witchcraft herself. (This was not as much of an issue in frontier Illinois as it would have been, say, a hundred and fifty years earlier in Massachusetts, but still, it wasn't something to brag about.) Nancy *had* to have known this was the most effective way to derail the relationship. She may not have realized the effect it would have on Rhoda – in fact, it is almost certain she didn't realize it until well after Rhoda's break.

Obviously, the entire Phenix family – most especially Charles and Nancy – immediately became personae non grata at the Derry cabin. Nancy was seen as the agent of Rhoda's misery. Charles may have been considered guilty by association. We'll never know, because Derry family history has given us only one side of the story. But no breakup is ever one-sided.

How did Charles react? It wasn't only Rhoda's hopes and dreams that were destroyed by Nancy's incantation. Charles' plans for his future with Rhoda came crashing down as well. If the situation had been different, maybe Charles and Rhoda could have made things work. If Nancy's threat of a curse hadn't taken hold of Rhoda's mind so firmly, maybe the young lovers could have worked through the dark times. They could have come out on the other side of the darkness still holding hands, battered and worn, but still together.

But that's not the way things happened.

We can imagine that Charles was very protective of Rhoda. She was the baby of her family. She was the girl he wanted to marry. In a small town on the frontier, Charles had made his choice – he had every intention of spending the rest of his life with Rhoda. He wouldn't have simply abandoned her. Nancy may have kept Charles away from Rhoda after the confrontation, but he was very likely still emotionally invested in the relationship.

Therefore, we can guess that maybe Charles shamed Nancy into trying to make amends.

Imagine an unimaginable situation: Charles is kept away from his intended bride, the love of his life, the girl he wants to marry and build a life with. He's not allowed to visit her, but he hears rumors in the community that horrible things are happening at the Derry house. Rhoda is losing her mind, and it's all Nancy Phenix's fault.

It must have taken all Charles' powers of persuasion to get Nancy to backpedal even as far as she did. She certainly never gave permission for the relationship to go forward, but she did at least try to convince Rhoda that there was no curse. Derry family lore gives us no indication of Nancy's state of mind when she attempted to see Rhoda. We will never know if Nancy actually did feel remorse over her actions, or if unpleasant town gossip nudged her to the Derry house, or if Charles finally wore her down.

In this effort of Nancy's to mend fences, there is never any mention of Charles. After he loses Rhoda, he simply disappears from Derry family oral tradition.

All of this, of course, is a boatload of what-ifs. We have absolutely no idea if any of this even happened. But maybe, just maybe, Charles was behind Nancy's attempted visit to Rhoda, the visit that failed so spectacularly. Maybe Charles fought back against his mother's decree. Maybe he shamed her into trying to make amends.

Maybe, Charles had nothing to do with Nancy's fruitless visit to Rhoda, to try to salvage the wreckage of the young woman's heart.

Or just maybe, he had everything to do with it.

All we know for sure is that Nancy's attempted apology came far too late to repair Rhoda's shattered sanity.

Whatever the depth of Charles' love for Rhoda, it would not be enough to save her. With her mental state deteriorating, Jacob and Rachel knew their daughter needed help – help they weren't trained to give her. Rhoda needed professional psychiatric help. The Derrys decided to commit Rhoda to the care of the doctors and nurses at the Illinois State Hospital for the Insane in Jacksonville, Illinois.

Sometime after 1856, when Rhoda was committed to Jacksonville, the Phenix family moved away from Ursa. Charles and his family disappear from the historical record after the heartwrenching debacle of 1852. The last time anything definite can be traced to them is when Nancy Phenix stopped Rhoda's brother in the street to try to apologize. After that, they're just ... gone.

There are several Charles Phenixes out there, Charles F. and Charles H. and Charles W., but none of them are our boy. If Nancy Phenix was embarrassed at her treatment of Rhoda, and its dreadful consequences, and wanted to fade into obscurity, she certainly got her wish.

And Charles? For now, Charles is nothing more than a ghost in the wind.

CHAPTER TEN
JACKSONVILLE

The mental health crusader Dorothea Dix wrote an impassioned plea to the Senate and House of Representatives of Illinois in January 1847. In this missive, she stated that in those modern times, insanity was no longer considered "the extinction of the mind". In the enlightened field of modern psychiatry, insanity was realized to be based on physical causes. These physical causes of lunacy could be treated successfully, just like any other disease.

Dix pointed out that the formation of an institution to care for the insane of Illinois wasn't just a generous thing to do – it was also a moral obligation. "Governments are bound ... to watch over, provide for, and protect certain classes, made dependent through the loss of various senses. Of such are the blind, the deaf and dumb, and most of all, the insane. All these require peculiar and various modes of care, differing so widely from the necessities of other classes in our communities, as to cast them absolutely on the charge of the State – a responsible and sacred trust."

What Dix really had in mind was an institution where the insane could be cured, if at all possible. Dix remarked that a Dr. Earle (of Bloomingdale Asylum in New York) wrote in his annual report of 1844 that with proper care, "where the proper measures are adopted in the early stages, no less than eighty in every hundred have been relieved ... there are few acute diseases from which so large a percentage of the persons attacked are restored, as from insanity." Aiming for an eighty percent cure rate was a lofty goal, but that's exactly what Dix had in mind.

Even the eminent Dr. Kirkbride, designer of asylums who gave his name to the Kirkbride style of building, agreed with this approach. Reporting from the Pennsylvania Hospital, he urged "early and prompt removal to suitable hospitals, by which large numbers are restored to health and usefulness in society, who otherwise would remain a burthen (sic) to themselves and their friends."

According to Dix (and several others, whom she quoted in her appeal to the Illinois Congress), it was a matter of simple economy. Treating insanity early, when there was a better chance of cure, was much less costly than caring for the incurable insane.

"Dr. Awl, of Ohio, records in 1842, that of twenty-five old cases, suffered to become incurable, the cost to the State and counties had already been $50,600; while twenty-five recent cases brought under seasonable treatment, had cost but $1,130; that is, $45.20 for each individual."

Why not let families care for their own insane at home? Dix had a rebuttal for that as well. "Recovery is so rare as it is nearly hopeless while the patient remains with his family, exposed to all the exciting causes which have developed the malady." Besides, Dix wrote, "the disturbances of the insane destroy all domestic order and business." Having an insane relative in your house disrupts home life, and that doesn't do anybody any good. Both the patient and her family suffer.

Dix had another motive in suggesting that Illinois build an institution for the care of the mentally ill. She was concerned about the mistreatment the insane were subjected to, if they were homeless and wandering around the countryside. "Again, of the insane who are regarded as harmless to themselves and others, and wander abroad, who has not witnessed the cruel persecutions by which they are often assailed on the part of thoughtless and idle men and boys?"

In response to Dix's eloquent plea, the state legislature decided to build a state hospital for the care of the mentally ill. The hospital, planned to be built just south of Jacksonville in Morgan County, adopted the plan of the Indiana State Hospital. As the hospital was originally designed to house two hundred and fifty patients and attendants, the Board of Trustees decided to use the Kirkbride plan, just in case they needed to go bigger in the future. (The Kirkbride asylum plan consisted of one big main building, with the capacity to attach two wings, one on either end. The wings could be further expanded outward as needed.)

The Illinois State Hospital for the Insane was established March 1, 1847, and construction began in 1848. Dix wanted to see the asylum opened by 1849, but it wasn't until November 3, 1851 that the first two wards were ready for occupants. The asylum was located on three hundred acres of land, on a spot with a reliable source of water and sufficient sources of fuel. The site was further developed into an idyllic landscape for the enjoyment of the future patients and staff. In March 1848, the steward bought 154 apple trees of different varieties from nurseries in Alton and St. Louis. One tree died, but the rest flourished in the orchard. From those same nurseries came seventy-one sugar maple trees, which the steward planted along the state road that ran past the hospital. He also planted elms and sycamores for shade.

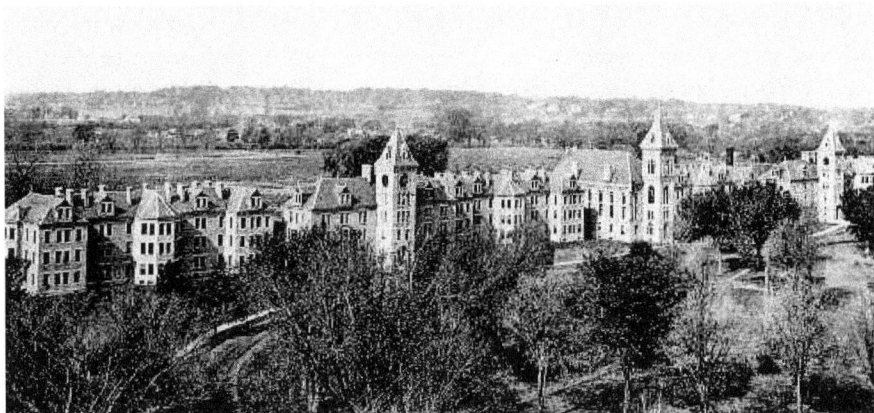

The Illinois State Hospital for the Insane in Jacksonville was opened to the first inmates in November 1851.

This frenzy of planting was done with the comfort and recreation of the patients in mind. In her recommendation for an asylum for Illinois, Dorothea Dix pointed to the examples set by the institutions in the east, particularly those in Vermont, Massachusetts, and Pennsylvania. These state hospitals had working farms, on which the patents were encouraged to help. This gave them something to occupy their time, and also helped offset the cost of food for the hospitals.

The state hospital was prepared to take in patients from every social class. Indigent patients were to be charged simply for the cost of their care, no more. Paying patients would be charged according to what the trustees thought was fair. And in considering patients for admittance, preference was to be given to the indigent of Illinois.

The Board of Trustees kept meticulous records for the first few years of the hospital's history, down to the pennies spent and to the last board-foot of black walnut used in the construction of the massive Kirkbride building. We can still read these records today, in an illuminating volume entitled *Reports of the Illinois State Hospital for the Insane, 1847-1862*. In addition to Dorothea Dix's eloquent letter to the Illinois legislature, the book contains nearly everything you'd ever want to know about the origins of the hospital at Jacksonville.

Far from being as dry as its title might suggest, the book makes for fascinating reading. To say the road to building the state hospital was rocky is putting it mildly. The members of the Board of Trustees for the early years of the hospital were an interesting bunch. They were – well, I don't want to say they were whiners, but by the time they wrote the Second Biennial Report, they were starting to get the idea that maybe it wasn't going to be so easy just to toss up a Kirkbride building and throw open the doors, welcoming the state's insane with open arms. Their best intentions notwithstanding, they soon realized there was more to putting an asylum together than they had first imagined.

The tone of the trustees' part of the Second Biennial Report has more than a touch of pique. "We at once enter upon ground over which the oldest and most civilized States have been compelled to feel their way, groping doubtfully and carefully, with many fears and many footfalls. How then shall we, a people of yesterday, expect to rear an asylum for our insane fellows up on the ground from which we have but just now frightened the panther and the prairie wolf, without unexpected delays and disappointments?"

Their main concern at that point in time was heating and ventilation. The board, over the course of two years of construction, had come to realize that heating a building three hundred feet long and fifty feet wide, housing two hundred to three hundred patients, "few of whom can be trusted with any possible access to fire", wasn't going to be so easy. They had to redesign the construction of flues as they went along. Simply putting a fireplace in every room was, of course, right out. The trustees had to decide, as the building was under construction, whether to heat the rooms with steam vents or with stoves. Plus, the contractor who had been hired to do all the brickwork completely flaked, and vanished halfway through the job. The board had to hire day laborers, and supervisors to watch them, to put up the walls.

To add to the board's embarrassment, the whole project was woefully over budget. When they'd started out, they had budgeted $60,000 to build an asylum for two hundred fifty patients plus their attendants. After that, someone read in the July 1849 report of the *American Journal of Insanity* that $60,000 was about as lowball as they could have gone. In fact, no institution of that size had been built for less than $250,000, except for the Ohio Asylum – which had cost $160,000. Even the Indiana State Hospital, which Jacksonville was modeled on, was still unfinished and could only serve sixty to seventy patients – and had already cost $70,000.

So the board decided they really needed at least $250,000, finally taking into account that labor and materials would cost more on the frontier. With a new budget in place, the board could turn to other matters, like exactly how to spend these new funds.

In contrast, Superintendent James M. Higgins wrapped up his part of the Second Biennial Report by assuring the trustees that three stories of the east wing would be built, heated, and roofed very soon, and that the west wing and center building would be completely finished by first of June, 1851. That date turned out to be a bit optimistic. The hospital wasn't ready for its first patient until early November 1851. The east wing would be ready to receive patients, Higgins said, as soon as possible.

Because of this enthusiasm for the project, we may forgive Superintendent Higgins the run-on sentence with which he closed his report. "With what commendable feelings of pride and pleasure must every philanthropic mind throughout our enterprising and prosperous State, contemplate the fact, that in so short a time, the means will be provided of administering relief to even a *part* of our unfortunate fellow citizens who are suffering from that most fearful of maladies – the malady of the mind; that the noble enterprise, set on foot by the enlightened and humane policy of the legislature, and kept alive and in motion by the liberality and benevolence of the great people they represent, is about to exert its power and efficacy in rescuing from the depths of wretchedness and woe, many a pitiable subject of insanity, now deprived of the aid and comfort he so much needs, and to furnish him a safe and comfortable retreat, where, in the midst of kind and attentive friends, his wants may be supplied, and his sorrows alleviated – where he may receive from the hands of his sympathizing physician, an anodyne for his pains, and the most efficient treatment, physical and moral, for the restoration of his disordered mind to its primitive condition of order and health."

The Illinois State Hospital for the Insane opened its doors on November 3, 1851. Sophronia McElhiney, of McLean County, was the first patient admitted.

In the Third Biennial Report, covering the years 1851 to 1852 – the first report filed after the opening of the hospital – the trustees started out by congratulating themselves, and they were right to do so. The project had been in the works for four years. The trustees admitted that at first they thought "with only two wards completed for either sex, with no possibility of proper classification, the noisy and the melancholy, the fastidious, the filthy, the obscene and even the idiotic, being all necessarily crowded together in the same wing", treatment of the insane was going to be difficult. They were, happily, mistaken. They pointed to the superintendent's report, which showed that even though the hospital took in a large number of chronic cases right away, thirty percent ended up cured.

The trustees did take the opportunity of their report that year to kvetch about the fact that a bill had passed in the Illinois legislature that reduced the number of trustees. The trustees were insulted by this, and they had every right to be. The reduction was snuck past, tacked onto another bill (one that established the Illinois Institution for the Education of the Blind). The trustees' ire was barely hidden by the professional, genteel nineteenth century language of the report. The trustees were feeling very put-upon, and it showed.

"Let it also be remembered that at the time this revolution was thus attempted, there was not even a pretended cause for it. The then-existing body of trustees were (sic) entirely harmonious among themselves ... the building in all its parts was progressing more rapidly and more satisfactorily to the State than it had ever been before, and the representatives of the people were not only willing to grant all the board asked of them but even more."

The board pointed out, quite sensibly, that whoever was responsible for reducing the number of trustees was sending the wrong message. The mentally ill needed stability above all, and their relatives needed to be reassured that the institution to which they committed their loved ones for care was being run properly and competently. The board used the third report to lash out at the state legislature, complaining bitterly about the unfair attacks on the hospital.

"Rumors have been circulated ... to produce the impression either that we were totally incompetent to our trusts, or actively abusing them. The superintendent has been represented as totally unfit for his duties – we have been charged with an extravagant and useless appropriation of rooms and of funds ... At one time our walls were about to fall down – at another our heating apparatus would certainly fail ... and no one ought to expect that the ship could be sailed successfully by such a crazy crew for a single week, even if successfully launched."

The board lashed out in defense: "We have called for a definite statement of the particular facts and cases in which either we or our officers have been in fault; but have received no reply ... We ask our opponents to point out to us and to the legislature the specific facts on which their charges are based, that if they exist they may be at once corrected or removed."

They saved their biggest dose of snark for the very end of the report. "It may be that all this is the result of mere accident, or magic, or miracle. It may be that the building sprung up on the prairie in spite of the incompetence of the superintendent and the board – and that the cures chanced, in spite of the ignorance of the officers who should have affected them. If so, such miracles will, probably, in due time, cease ... and then it will be fairly open to an honorable and successful attack. We maintain that, till that time, it is better still to trust to the same accident or magic which has, as a matter of fact, carried the institution safely so far rather than throw it into the arms of those who have done the best and worst they could to prevent and defeat these auspicious results." The reader can almost taste the bitter sarcasm that drips from the page.

In his part of the Third Biennial Report, Superintendent Higgins stayed away from politics, preferring instead to stick to a medically-based report. He explained the character of the first patients to be admitted. He wrote that the friends and families of many of the patients, hearing that the asylum was nearing completion, deluged the institution with urgent requests to have their relatives accepted into the asylum's care. This resulted in nearly all of the early patients admitted as being chronic and incurable cases.

This was, unfortunately, not the stated aim of the Illinois State Hospital. The asylum at Jacksonville was designed for the care of patients who would eventually get better, and be able to rejoin society. It wouldn't be until 1902, with the opening of the Illinois Asylum for the Incurable Insane (later known as the Peoria State Hospital), that an asylum would be dedicated to the care of chronic cases.

Dr. Higgins wrote that there were some patients who were noisy at night and disturbed the others. Those patients, he said, would be better off if they were kept at the outside end of the wing. This was the beginning of the hospital staff attempting to separate the patients according to their habits, trying to keep those who were violent away from those who were quieter in their insanity. The Eighth Ward would later be set aside for disturbed patients.

Dr. Higgins also included a list of "Supposed Causes of Insanity" as it pertained to the early patients at the hospital. This list was compiled from reports given by the friends and family of the patients, who admittedly were not expert diagnosticians. There were three women and seven men who suffered from "disappointed love", according to Dr. Higgins. Other causes of insanity in the Third Biennial Report included "injury of head" (four men, one woman), "study of scriptures" (one man), "intemperance" (again, one man), "intense study" (four men), "mental anxiety" (one man, three women), "jealousy" (a woman), and "lactation" (a woman … obviously). Interestingly, there is a distinction made between "study of scriptures", "intense study", "religious excitement", and "spiritual rappings".

Rhoda would have been mentioned in the Fifth and Sixth Biennial Reports – mostly the sixth. The fifth report was published in December 1856, soon after her arrival. The sixth would have covered the years 1856 to 1858, which is when Rhoda would have been living there. The records mention that twelve women from Adams County had been admitted since December 1, 1854. By the time of the Fifth Biennial Report, Dr. Andrew McFarland was the superintendent, having replaced Dr. Higgins. In the "Table of Alleged Causes of Insanity", Rhoda may have been lumped in with the seven patients suffering from "disappointed affection" (although the cause directly above this on the list, "menstrual irregularities", from which eight women suffered, was mentioned years later as Rhoda's affliction). Other causes listed in the table for 1856 included "hard study", "abuse of opium", "vicious indulgences", "injury of head", "sudden accession of fortune", and "excessive use of tobacco".

Today, we find some of these reasons backward and utterly laughable. We congratulate ourselves for being so modern that "religious excitement" is no longer a reason to commit someone to a mental hospital. But even in the middle of the nineteenth century, some physicians and psychiatrists were beginning to challenge the old ways of looking at mental illness. In this report, Dr. McFarland wrote, "The causes of insanity, as they may appear in such a document as this, are usually looked for with especial attention ... The usual routine of causes, which, time out of mind, have served to fill out a tabular statement, have long been considered ... extremely unsatisfactory. Yet it is difficult for popular sentiment, or even for science itself, to become divested of the old and easy belief, that insanity ... will observe the mathematical sequence of a problem in proportion."

McFarland went on to say that really, if you think about it, the root causes of insanity are so complex that it's quite hubristic of doctors to point to one underlying cause of insanity per person. Furthermore, he said, treatment of insanity isn't as easy as treating what seems to be the main cause of the mania. "This would be so," he wrote, "if the relations of cause and effect were always calculable."

McFarland was advanced enough in his theories to realize this wasn't always the case. Take the person suffering from "religious mania". Maybe this person had a family history of insanity, but his particular mania manifested itself in religious experience. "The case is committed to us as one unquestionably caused by 'religious excitement'. Yet nothing can be less conclusive. The religious cast infused into all the outward manifestations of the insanity is simply accidental."

Dr. Andrew McFarland's appointment as superintendent at Jacksonville marked the starting point of the modern era of the care of the insane in Illinois. He served for fifteen years, from 1854 to 1869, and his ideas formed the foundation of modern psychiatric care.

Dr. McFarland was violently opposed to patient restraint. He pointed out that in a large institution, perhaps only one-fourth of the patients actually needed to be restrained – but care was dictated by the weakest link. "For those who do not need [restraint], the bolts and bars found in all our asylums are not only no advantage, they are positively injurious. They irritate many patients and retard their recovery."

He was among the first to suggest that patients be given jobs to keep them occupied during the day, and he was able to implement that at Jacksonville. He also wanted to run the hospital on a cottage system, with forty patients to each house, but the Kirkbride building had already been built. So, unlike Dr. Zeller fifty years later at the Peoria State Hospital, Dr. McFarland had to settle for what he'd been given.

No matter its rocky beginnings, the state hospital was by far the best option for Rhoda's care in her early insanity. In the early 1850s, the hospital at Jacksonville was state of the art, brand new and built to the most modern specifications. It had farms, shade trees, and an orchard for the enjoyment of the patients. (The hospital did have to rebuild its barn fairly soon after it opened. On July 22, 1852, a patient, who had previously been calm enough not to be constantly watched by an attendant, set fire to the barn, which burned to the ground.)

All patients were encouraged to help out around the hospital and its grounds. Male patients tended vegetables in the gardens, sawed lumber, and pumped water into the tanks which supplied the baths and water closets. Female patients made clothing and other cloth goods (tablecloths, carpets, curtains, bags for hams) for the hospital. In 1852, they even helped to sew twelve straitjackets.

The staff of the hospital was extremely well trained for the time – or at least, the superintendent and matron were supposed to hold them to a very high code of conduct. The first and most important rule was to be kind. "The attendant should consider the patient as his honored guest, who comes, tarries for a short season, and goes on his way ... patients should always be greeted ... [and] should always be addressed in courteous language, and never be made subject to any opprobrious epithet or nick-name."

Attendants were expected to be above reproach in their personal habits. Anyone known to be a drinker or gambler wasn't hired. Employees were discouraged from gossiping about the asylum's patients, whether at work or outside the hospital. The staff was urged to treat the patients with "unvarying kindness". They were not allowed to yell across the wards at a patient. Anyone heard taunting or threatening a patient was summarily fired. The same went for physical abuse. "A blow, kick, or any other form of physical abuse inflicted on a patient, will be sufficient reason for the prompt dismissal of the individual so offending."

The attendants were also not allowed to use any more force than was necessary in their handling of the patients in their care. "Attendants are considered, in this institution, the guardians and companions, but not the 'keepers' of the patients." The staff was responsible for keeping the patients mentally engaged and entertained.

And they were held to that standard constantly. "The attendants' place of duty is on the wards with their patients. During duty hours, and while the patients are out of their sleeping apartments, they have no business in their own rooms ... and any attendant discovered in his or her room engaged in reading, writing, playing on any instrument of music, entertaining visitors, or otherwise off duty, is acting in violation of rule."

Similarly, the attendants were encouraged to get outside with patients for fresh air, but not to abuse the privilege. "Attendants are forbidden to make walking out with their patients a pretext of doing errands or making calls for themselves."

The staff was responsible for daily care of the patients, making sure they were clean and dressed each day, and that the wards were tidy. Male patients were shaved every Wednesday and Saturday, and patients' hair and nails were trimmed on a regular basis. Patients got tepid baths once a week. "It is highly desirable that the feet be washed, even when general bathing is not possible."

Mealtimes were genteel affairs as well. The attendants dined with the patients, and the staff was not allowed to hurry the patients through their meals. Rather, they were allowed to eat at their leisure. "Habits in eating differ, and all – the old particularly – should have time to protract their eating to full extent." It was all very civilized – except for the rule that "after each meal the knives and forks shall be counted before being taken away from the table".

The asylum was very conscientious about not wasting food. Perhaps this was a reaction to the very early days of being drastically over-budget. "Food that may have been handled, or rendered unfit for eating, should be sent back to a receptacle of its own, but whatever is fit to be served in another form should be carefully laid by itself for future consumption."

The evening hours were designed to be just as relaxing. One attendant was present at all times on each ward after lights out. "Should a patient, after retiring, call for water, as will often be the case, or for any aid within the attendant's power, it should be immediately supplied."

There were strict instructions, in the staff handbook, for the night watchman's duty. "His first duty shall be to attend to the security of the door-fastenings and the safe condition of all places where fire has been used during the day." Any unusual circumstances were to be reported to the superintendent in the morning.

That's worth repeating: "Should anything unusual attract his attention ... he shall call the notice of the proper attendant to it." Because here's where Rhoda's story gets *really* weird.

I cannot explain what happened to Rhoda Derry while she was in the state hospital at Jacksonville. I can only write it down.

The procedure for admitting someone to the state hospital in the mid-nineteenth century seems crude to us today. For one thing, it was much more involved than simply taking someone to the hospital. "Some respectable person" living in the same county as the prospective patient had to file a statement with the judge of the county court naming two witnesses, one of whom had to be a doctor. Then the clerk of the court issued a subpoena for the witnesses. They would appear in court and testify, along with six subpoenaed jurors (again, one of the jurors had to be a physician). The verdict of insanity was written up and presented to the board of trustees by the clerk of the court. The superintendent was, ultimately, the person who decided if the hospital could receive the patient. If so, he told the clerk to issue a warrant for the sheriff to arrest the insane person and bring him to the hospital.

This was undoubtedly a traumatic experience. For Rhoda, who was battling imaginary witches and who just wanted to be left alone to mourn Charles, it must have been devastating. Rhoda was a young woman, only twenty-two when she was committed. If she had any sense of what was happening to her at all, she must have been furiously embarrassed at being arrested and taken to a mental hospital.

Rhoda may have been admitted to the Eighth Ward, which was reserved for severely disturbed patients. The Eighth Ward was the only ward on which straitjackets were used. It also contained the "screen" room, a cell-like bedroom that had locked screens over the window and door. In accordance with hospital policy, Rhoda was locked in her room every night.

And every morning, she was found wandering the grounds of the hospital.

When she was found, the harried attendant would ask Rhoda who let her out of her locked room. The answer Rhoda gave was always the same.

"Nancy Phenix let me out."

Was Rhoda simply seeing things that weren't there? Could this have been a visual hallucination, similar to the terrors she experienced before she even came to Jacksonville?

But if this was just a hallucination, how do we explain the unlocked door? Was this nightly visitor a spirit? Was it some entity that Rhoda's mind interpreted as Nancy Phenix? Rhoda didn't keep a journal, so we have no idea what form her scattered thoughts took. And the attendants at the hospital, as kind as they may have been, were not prepared to believe the ramblings of an insane young woman.

Even now, one hundred and sixty years after Rhoda Derry spent time at the hospital in Jacksonville, the singular mystery of her experience there remains. Rhoda's nightly encounters with the entity she called Nancy Phenix are just one more inexplicable part of her story.

The staff of the hospital was never able to explain this bizarre state of affairs. It remains part of Rhoda's mystery to this day.

By the time of the Fourth Biennial Report (December 1, 1854), the superintendent and board of trustees had admitted that while the Illinois State Hospital for the Insane was indeed designed as a "hospital" to cure insanity, there were some of their patients who were incurable. The board seems to have struggled with this concept, and with good reason. They realized almshouses were a natural dumping ground for the incurable insane. Remember, the asylum at Bartonville wouldn't exist for another fifty years.

Almshouses were, on the whole, dismal failures at caring for the harmless but incurable insane. The board sincerely felt that the insane should either be cared for by their family, or secluded in properly run asylums, like the one at Jacksonville. The staff was justifiably proud of their hospital, and worked very hard to keep it healthful, useful, and above all, accountable to the public.

As Dr. Andrew McFarland put it, "...the number in our charge has increased to a point where the curative efficiency of our institution is in danger of being impaired by the crowded condition of its apartments." The hospital was equipped to care for two hundred patients – they regularly had over two hundred and fifty. At that point, the asylum was using dayrooms, originally intended for recreation and socialization, as dormitories. They simply didn't have enough space for their patients.

At the same time, the board of trustees wanted to help as many of the insane of Illinois as they could. They could best do that, they decided, by sending the incurables home to their families. State law required a two-year observation period to decide if a patient was curable or not. If a patient hadn't shown at least some improvement at the end of two years, according to the board of trustees, they were sent home as incurable. This is what happened to Rhoda Derry.

The procedure for when a patient was discharged was fairly similar to intake procedure. The superintendent told the county clerk for the patient's home county that he or she was ready to be discharged. The clerk issued another warrant to the sheriff, who came to the hospital and transported the patient back home.

Rhoda wasn't alone in the misery she faced in her time at Jacksonville. Just a few years later, the Illinois State Hospital for the Insane would be home to a woman whose story was almost as strange as Rhoda's ... but with a very different ending.

CHAPTER ELEVEN
ELIZABETH PACKARD

Elizabeth Parsons Ware, born in 1816, was raised in a home where she was encouraged to learn, and to speak her own mind. Even in Massachusetts, this was unusual for girl children in the early nineteenth century. But Elizabeth was a daughter of a minister, so she got the benefit of schooling, and of listening to her father's discussions with other learned men. Elizabeth's outspokenness attracted the attention of Theophilus Packard, a fellow minister and friend of the Ware family. Theophilus and Elizabeth were married May 21, 1839, despite the groom being fourteen years older than the bride. The couple settled in Manteno, in Kankakee County, Illinois, and had six children.

Elizabeth was intelligent and well-spoken, good attributes for a minister's wife. But twenty years into their marriage, the cracks began to show.

Theophilus had very rigidly held religious beliefs, including strict ideas on the raising of children. Elizabeth was torn at the sight of one of her young sons in tears because his father had hinted that maybe the kid just wasn't *good* enough to get into Heaven. Elizabeth was incensed at the Calvinist belief that an innocent child could be found unworthy of a heavenly reward, and she started telling people about her reservations.

To have a woman voicing independent thought was bad enough, but Elizabeth was soon arguing church doctrine with her husband, who, being a minister, was not pleased. Even worse, she was questioning Reverend Packard's beliefs in front of members of the congregation. The couple argued about other things too, like family finances, child rearing, and the issue of slavery. But the issue of religion was the most divisive. Theophilus couldn't stand the fact that Elizabeth so freely expressed religious opinions that were contrary to his own.

When the state hospital opened at Jacksonville in 1851, the state legislature passed a law outlining the procedures for committal. Rhoda Derry would have been allowed a public hearing before being committed, even against her will. Everyone got their day in court. However, there was an exception to this law: a husband could have his wife committed without her consent, and without a public hearing. This law was ostensibly written that way for the sake of protecting children in the family who might be in danger from a violently insane mother, the caregiver. But Theophilus saw a way out of the embarrassment of having an outspoken wife.

Theophilus Packard decided that Elizabeth was "slightly insane". Conscious of the need for witnesses, he invited a doctor, J. W. Brown, to the house to interview her. Dr. Brown arrived incognito, pretending to be a sewing machine salesman. During their conversation, Elizabeth opened up to her visitor, complaining that her husband dominated her, and saying he told people she was insane. Dr. Brown promptly turned around and reported all of this to Theophilus, along with the observation that Elizabeth "exhibited a great dislike to me". Maybe Elizabeth found the "sewing machine salesman" cover story a little dodgy. The end result was that Theophilus decided to have Elizabeth committed.

Elizabeth learned of this decision on June 18, 1860, when the county sheriff arrived at the Packard home to take her into custody. She did not go quietly; she made the sheriff and his assistant carry her to the train.

She spent three years at the state hospital in Jacksonville. She spent the entire time writing letters to friends, begging them for help in getting released. She steadfastly refused to agree that she was insane, or to change her religious views.

She raised such a fuss that in January 1864, she was finally brought to Kankakee City for a jury trial. In front of Judge Charles Starr, Theophilus's relatives testified that Elizabeth had argued with her husband and tried to leave his congregation. They agreed with Theophilus that, clearly, this was a sign of insanity.

Elizabeth's lawyers, Stephen Moore and John W. Orr, responded by calling their own witnesses – people from the neighborhood who knew the Packards but were not members of Theophilus's church. These people testified they had never seen any sign of insanity in Elizabeth's behavior, or in her conversations with them, whether she was discussing religion or just chatting about the weather. The final witness called was Dr. Duncanson, who was both a physician and a theologian. He said, while he didn't necessarily agree with every one of Elizabeth's religious beliefs, "I do not call people insane because they differ with me."

The jury took seven minutes to decide in Elizabeth's favor.

Judge Starr declared Elizabeth Packard to be legally sane, and issued an order that she be released. She was discharged from the state hospital as "incurable". When Elizabeth returned to her home in Manteno, she found that

Theophilus had rented out their house, sold her furniture, and the night before her release, had taken her money, her clothes, and the children and moved to Boston.

Elizabeth moved back in with her parents temporarily, but she still burned for independence – and she wanted to get her children back. She decided that, to support herself, she would write a book about her experiences, as a cautionary tale for others. In November 1860, she had published a pamphlet entitled "Reproof to Dr. McFarland for His Abuses of His Patients" (which did not endear her to the higher-ups at the state hospital). It cost her $100 to print up a thousand pamphlets, which she sold for ten cents each, netting $90 in profit. If she could sell a pamphlet, she figured, why not try selling a book?

The printer told her that the cost of printing a thousand copies of a book would come to $2500. It was pricey, but Elizabeth wasn't discouraged. One night, as she was getting ready for bed, she had a brainstorm – she would sell promissory notes for fifty cents each, which could be redeemed for books when she got the book written and published. This would give her enough for a down payment to the printer. She also realized her readers would be more likely to redeem a ticket they'd already bought, than follow up on a nebulous promise to buy a book when it came out.

Elizabeth soon had her routine established. She would roll into town on the train. Her first stop would be the local hotel, where she would make her base. She would find a "reliable agent" – usually the town postmaster or a bookseller – who would agree to store the books when they arrived, and would deliver them to the ticket holders. Then she would canvass the town, selling tickets everywhere.

This determination propelled Elizabeth Packard through the eventual publication of four books. She first wrote *Marital Power Exemplified, or Three Years Imprisoned for Religious Belief* (1864). She followed that with *Great Disclosure of Spiritual Wickedness in High Places* (1865), *The Mystic Key or The Asylum Secret Unlocked* (1866), and *The Prisoners' Hidden Life, or Insane Asylums Revealed* (1868). Along with her writing career, she gained renown as a speaker, and worked tirelessly to change laws regarding the treatment of the insane – and those who were merely accused of insanity.

On March 5, 1867, Illinois passed the Bill for the Protection of Personal Liberty. The bill was the result of Elizabeth's campaigning, and it guaranteed all people accused of insanity, including wives, the right to a public hearing. The wording was very specific, and there was a dig at Jacksonville (and obliquely, at Dr. McFarland). Given the tussling back and forth between the hospital and the state legislature fifteen years before, I wonder if the specific mention of the state hospital was on purpose.

"No superintendent, medical director, agent or other person, having the management, supervision or control of the Insane Hospital at Jacksonville, or of any hospital or asylum for insane and distracted persons in this State, shall receive, detain or keep in custody at such asylum or hospital any person who has not been declared insane or distracted by a verdict of a jury and the order of a court."

Elizabeth Ware Packard's campaigning in states all over the country led to reform in commitment and treatment procedures. Some reports credit her with getting as many as thirty-four laws changed in Illinois, Iowa, and Massachusetts. Most of the legislation involved changes in the requirements for committal, in particular, mandatory jury trials for those accused of being insane. No longer could a husband put his wife away without a trial.

Elizabeth had mixed feelings toward Dr. McFarland, to say the least. As the superintendent at the state hospital, McFarland was at the top of the list of people Elizabeth blamed for her wrongful committal. She knew she wasn't insane. Why couldn't this educated doctor – the guy in charge – realize it as well?

Elizabeth's attitude toward McFarland vacillated between irritation at her committal, and, oddly, a type of hero worship. Elizabeth even wrote an extremely ill-advised letter to McFarland, expressing her admiration for him, and telling him she hoped they could be partners after death in a heavenly marriage. (Equally ill-advisedly, McFarland kept the letter, which honestly didn't look good for either one of them.)

We shouldn't fall into the trap of blaming Dr. McFarland right along with Elizabeth. He felt just as strongly as she did about the procedure of committal. Two years before Mrs. Packard's trial, Dr. McFarland felt it necessary to write in the Eighth Biennial Report (1862) something about the method of committing a patient to an asylum. He recognized the seriousness of having someone committed: "It must be remembered that the act implies something more than simply placing an individual under particular medical advice and treatment. It involves a deprivation of personal liberty ... Like the suspension of *habeas corpus*, it is an absolute seizure of the rights of man, which only the gravest necessities can justify." This was a doctor who was absolutely *not* cavalier about the rights of the insane.

Dr. McFarland implored those considering committing their loved one to the Illinois State Hospital not to use any deception. "Inform him candidly and without disguise, that, by a common agreement among his best friends, he is to be placed for a while in the Hospital ... The complaint is almost daily heard here; 'I can forgive them everything else except their deceiving me!'"

This was written at the end of 1862, when Elizabeth Packard had been at the state hospital for a year and a half. She was no doubt one of the patients from whom Dr. McFarland heard that very same "complaint"! She had every reason to feel helpless and deceived. Her husband had faked her out with a doctor disguised as a sewing machine salesman. So why did McFarland ignore her, when she was so obviously not insane?

The reason may have been that Elizabeth was distraught when she first came to the hospital, and it's possible she made a bad first impression. She had every reason to be upset. She'd been torn from her six children, the youngest of whom was still a toddler. Knowing Theophilus's ideas on child rearing, she feared for her children's welfare and emotional health. (She was right to fear – her youngest daughter was saddled with the care of a household of seven people when she was still a gradeschooler. The responsibility damaged the girl beyond repair, and she died young, a raving maniac in her thirties.)

After Elizabeth calmed down somewhat, she made the best of a bad situation by taking charge of the ward in which she lived. She cleaned the rooms along with the attendants, and encouraged the insane patients to get outside for fresh air. She also had conversations with Dr. McFarland as often as she could manage. And yet, she wrote a pamphlet in November 1860, when she'd been at the hospital five months, attacking McFarland for abuses of his patients.

It's possible there was some weird dynamic going on, some love/hate relationship neither Elizabeth nor Dr. McFarland would admit to, something neither of them could explain. It would have been so easy for McFarland to throw out the bizarre letter Elizabeth wrote to him. But he didn't. He kept it long after she had been discharged – with a diagnosis of incurably insane. It's also strange that Dr. McFarland kept Elizabeth at the hospital for three years, when the regulations said that a patient, if not cured, should be discharged as incurable after an observation period of two years.

The Illinois State Hospital at Jacksonville was not a horrible place. On the contrary, its superintendents and trustees held their staff to the highest of standards. The hospital was the most modern institution for the care of the insane yet seen in Illinois. It was wonderful for those suffering from a temporary state of insanity.

But the hospital's care failed both Rhoda Derry and Elizabeth Ware Packard. It failed Elizabeth, of course, because she wasn't insane. She was just put away by her husband, as a way to get rid of her. (This was vindictive, yes, but also rather shortsighted of Theophilus, as the state hospital was not a long-term care facility. He should have known she would eventually be discharged, even if she was discharged as incurable. Theophilus Packard, and the legislature of Illinois, turned out to have a tiger by the tail in Elizabeth.)

And the Illinois State Hospital failed Rhoda Derry, too. By the time she was admitted, it was too late for her. She was too broken even then for the staff to fix.

CHAPTER TWELVE
LIFE AFTER JACKSONVILLE

Rhoda was admitted to the state hospital at Jacksonville in 1856, and released sometime in 1858. Her condition was deemed incurable, and she was returned to her parents in Lima.

Rhoda seemed to have calmed down just a little after her discharge from the Illinois State Hospital. Derry family history doesn't mention any recurrence of Rachel shooting at imaginary witches in the house after Rhoda's return. But the random weirdness of life with Rhoda continued.

Rhoda was released from the asylum as incurable. A newspaper article, published in the *Quincy Daily Journal* on November 23, 1906, gives more information. Levi P. Slater, son of Anderson and Mary Jane (Derry) Slater, wrote a letter to Dr. Zeller when he heard of his Aunt Rhoda's passing. He wrote: "When the keeper of the asylum brought her back ... he did not know what was the matter with her. She was like the man referred to in the New Testament, who lived among the tombs."

Levi's stories continued. "Not long after Rhoda returned home, she ran to her bed and turned a somersault and lit on the bed on her head and whirled about like a top, with her feet straight up in the air. Her brother, Jerimiah, ran to her bedroom to see what the matter was and upon seeing Rhoda said, 'What are you doing? Get down from that bed.' Rhoda declared, 'I cannot, they are holding me.' Jerimiah asked, 'Who is holding you?' Rhoda replied, 'I do not know.'"

One very cold night, Rhoda's sister, Mary Jane, was home for a family visit with her husband, Anderson Slater. Andy slept on a cot near Rhoda's bed, because Rachel feared that Rhoda would kick off her covers during the night and shiver her way to wakefulness. It was Andy's duty to make sure Rhoda was covered with blankets that cold night. During the night, Andy had a strange dream – a black cat came into the house and ran around on the ceiling three times, then jumped on his face and scratched him.

In the morning, he told Rhoda about his dream. She said, "I dreamed the same thing" – then gasped when she got a good look at his face.

Scratches, as if from the claws of a cat, burned and throbbed on Anderson's face.

Another time, Rhoda, Andy and Mary Jane were all out in the yard. Rhoda grew very agitated, and asked Andy to climb the old elm tree that stood in the yard and plug up a hole in the tree. If he didn't, Rhoda said, a terrible wind would spring up. Andy refused, pointing out that it was a beautiful day, with not a breath of wind. Rhoda begged him to climb the tree, saying, "Please, hurry, the wind is coming." Mary Jane muttered to her husband, "Just do it – maybe she'll see that she is being silly."

Andy shrugged, and began to climb the tree. As he got higher and higher, the branches began to toss fitfully. Soon the tree was whipping in the gusts of a powerful wind, nearly knocking Anderson from his perch. But people in the house below were completely unaware that there was any wind blowing.

"Many other remarkable things occurred during Rhoda's early insanity," the article continued. "She frequently used large words, and properly, too, although she had never had an opportunity of acquiring an education."

Some of Rhoda's antics weren't as innocuous as using fifty cent words. Rhoda didn't acquire any tools for self-care during her stay in Jacksonville. She didn't know how to quiet her sometimes dangerous mind. The specter of Nancy Phenix still plagued her. "Sometimes she would say she saw Mrs. Phenix in the bed and she would butt her head against the door and imagine she was fighting the witches."

One of the weirdest stories from this period of Rhoda's life concerns her newly-acquired gift for telling the future. Jacob and Jerimiah went into town to get supplies. While they were there, Jacob sent Jerry to the post office to pick up the family's mail.

Meanwhile, at home, Rhoda told her mother, "Basil and Fredericka are coming for a visit." (Basil was Rhoda's second-oldest brother, and Fredericka was his second wife.) When Rachel asked Rhoda how she knew this, Rhoda couldn't tell her, but added that the couple had news of a new baby. That night, when Jacob and Jerimiah returned from their trip to town, Jacob told Rachel they'd gotten a letter from Basil. Jerry read the letter aloud. Basil and Fredericka would be arriving the following week, and they had news to share. When the couple came for their visit, Basil announced that Fredericka was expecting a child. She gave birth to Matilda Elsie, the couple's third child, in 1858.

On another occasion, a stranger came to the Derry home. Rhoda asked him for a chaw of tobacco. (She had picked up the habit in her teens.) When he gave it to her, she told him his name and what he wanted of her father. This information, coming as it did out of nowhere, flustered the man so badly that he climbed back on his horse and left at a fast gallop.

This incident brings up an interesting question. Moll Derry was renowned for her fortune-telling skills. If she was in a good mood, and got her offering of coffee, all was well. It may have been unconscious, but Rhoda seems almost to have been channeling Moll's abilities and her theatrics. It's said psychic talent is hereditary, and sometimes it can skip a generation. We have no evidence that Jacob had any psychic leanings, or that he even had any interest in carrying on his mother's practice of hex magic.

Rhoda may have inherited her grandmother's psychic abilities. But coupled with her mental illness, those abilities were warped. Maybe it was something in her delivery, but people weren't impressed with Rhoda's fortune-telling skills. They were just really disconcerted – even scared.

This was not a case of dementia praecox or epilepsy. I don't think Rhoda's mental illness stemmed from any organic cause. After the confrontation with Nancy Phenix, Rhoda's troubles, although they were very real, had a decidedly supernatural flavor to them. I think that Mollie Derry had more of an influence on Rhoda than anyone imagined.

What did Jacob and Rachel think when their youngest daughter came home from the asylum still broken?

The Derrys were poor farmers, not well educated folks. In an earlier time, they might have interpreted Rhoda's troubles as actual witchcraft. Even as things stood, either one of them could have whispered "witchcraft" in the private corners of their mind, in the darkest hours of the night. Jacob's own mother was both respected and feared for her magickal abilities, which sometimes skated dangerously close to the occult. Both Jacob and Rachel had memories of Moll's hex magic practice. This could have colored their thoughts, to be sure.

But Rhoda was their cherished daughter. It must have been a wrench for the whole family when Rhoda was returned to them from the asylum, dismissed as "incurable". No parent wants to hear that about their child.

We don't know what kind of social life Jacob and Rachel had, but when Rhoda's troubles began, it's likely the family became socially isolated. What friends they did have probably drifted away – either they were scared off by Rhoda's bizarre behavior, or they got tired of listening to Jacob and Rachel talk about their daughter's affliction. We do know that Rhoda's antics in the years between 1858 and 1860 were legitimately weird. News travels fast in a small town. People could have been so freaked out by Rhoda's strangeness that they just stopped visiting, effectively shunning the Derrys altogether. That can only have increased the sense of isolation Jacob and Rachel felt.

CHAPTER THIRTEEN
DESCENT INTO DARKNESS

Late summer, 1860. In farming communities, this was haying time, one of the busiest times of the year. But in the Derry household, there was no one to send the workers off to the fields, no one to bring sweating pitchers of lemonade or switchel to the men working under the sweltering sun to bring in the hay.

Rachel Derry had died.

Rachel Bright Derry seems to have been the only person who really understood Rhoda's mental illness. When Rhoda would cower in terror on the floor, whimpering that "witches" were after her, Rachel would load a pistol and shoot into the air to drive them off. She understood her daughter's affliction – or if she didn't understand it, she was willing to indulge it.

Rachel died sometime after the information for the 1860 census was collected. When she did, Rhoda lost her ally. It's not that Jacob loved his daughter any less than Rachel did. Jacob just lacked a mother's touch. Jacob buried his wife in Tioga Cemetery, four short miles from Lima, in Hancock County, just three-quarters of a mile north of the Adams-Hancock county line. Then he turned his attention to Rhoda.

In August of 1860, Jacob and Rachel, along with Rhoda, were living with the Jacobs family. According to the 1860 census, the people in the household were James C. Jacobs, aged 32 (a master cooper), his wife Elizabeth S. Jacobs, aged 27, and their young son Morris, who was seven years old. Jacob (listed as a "laborer") and Rachel were also in the house, as well as Rhoda, who was 25 at the time.

Joan Brown Derry, who has done extensive genealogy research on her family, has an interesting take on the situation.

> "I wondered why Jacob, Rachel, and Rhoda (already insane) were living with a Jacobs family in the 1860 Illinois Census. Had they lost their home? Who were the Jacobs in relationship to the Derrys? There were never any clues to these questions. Then I read about the laws in Illinois and the poor. It

said the following: 'Public care of the poor in Illinois began in 1819. In that year the General Assembly passed a law mandating public care and maintenance of those unable to support themselves and without family support. County Overseers of the poor farmed out care of the destitute to private caregivers.' (*Laws of Illinois 1819, p. 127*)

"I wonder if the elderly Jacob and Rachel (ages 65 and 63) with an insane daughter, couldn't manage any more on their own and applied to the county commissioners for assistance? If so, I wonder if they were 'farmed-out' to the Jacobs family for maintenance and support reasons?"

So Jacob was mourning his wife, who had just died relatively young. And living in someone else's home, with an insane daughter to care for, can't have been easy on   anyone involved.

We don't know if Elizabeth Jacobs required Rhoda to help with any chores around the house. But one thing is certain – even if she'd been asked, Rhoda was not capable of even the simplest household work. She didn't have the patience to bend scrubbing over a washtub on laundry day. She didn't have the patience to stand outside at the clothesline, snapping the dresses to get the wrinkles out, smoothing the pants, lining up the towels before pegging them to the line. She didn't have the patience to stand at a kitchen table kneading bread until it was as smooth and plump as a baby's bottom, then tuck it into a loaf pan ready for the oven.

Rhoda wasn't capable of doing any of the boring, repetitive tasks that were required of a farm woman on the Illinois frontier. Eggs would go ungathered if left to Rhoda's care, or get smashed against the henhouse wall if she succumbed to one of her fits of rage. A nervous cow wouldn't stand still to be milked. And Rhoda certainly wasn't up to the more perilous chores, like baking with a wood-fired stove, dipping candles into hot wax for hours at a time, or stirring a pot full of boiling lye to make soap.

We don't know if Rhoda had the ability, or even the desire, to help in her own recovery. That first blow, losing Charles in such a dramatic way, plus being held in Jacksonville for two years, may have simply broken her spirit beyond all hope of repair.

Was Rhoda still mourning the loss of Charles after all that time? Or had her personality warped into something darker, more savage? Did the shock of that early loss shatter her psyche, letting other pathologies – paranoia, anxiety, violence – slither through the cracks?

Whatever the cause of Rhoda's troubles, we do know that after Rachel's death, Jacob was no longer able to keep Rhoda in the home in which the family was boarding. The request of the County Overseer notwithstanding, James and Elizabeth Jacobs may have insisted Rhoda be removed from their home. Perhaps, without Rachel's calming influence on Rhoda, they may have feared for their young son's safety.

So Jacob made the heart-wrenching decision to have Rhoda committed to the Adams County almshouse.

Rhoda had already been institutionalized once. She spent two years at the state hospital in Jacksonville. Why didn't Jacob send her back there, where she could be cared for properly, by doctors and attendants trained in the treatment of the mentally ill? Why was Rhoda not allowed to go back to Jacksonville in 1860?

The reason was simple: the state hospital at Jacksonville wouldn't have taken her. She had been released in 1858, two years before, as incurable. Not only that, the state hospital was not equipped to handle a case like Rhoda's. The Illinois State Asylum in Jacksonville was not designed as a long-term care facility. Their beds were only available for a limited time. Their job was to care for the mentally ill and coax them back to health. If that took six months, wonderful. That patient was released, and another took their place. Over the course of, say, five years, ten patients could be helped (assuming an average stay of six months). And this was an ongoing process. An incurable patient, if allowed to stay, would have taken up that bed for decades. The staff would have had to focus their resources on just one patient instead of the dozens who could have circulated through the asylum in the same amount of time. If a patient didn't recover within two years, that was it – they'd had their chance. It was time to let someone else occupy that bed and benefit from the attentions of the staff.

In a large, boisterous family, the children tend to band together, in a sort of "us against the world" bond of solidarity. A triumph for one is a shared triumph; a slight against one is an injury to all. The bond between siblings, if they're close, can be very strong, lasting a lifetime.

When their baby sister found someone to love, Rhoda's brothers and sisters must have been overjoyed. 1850 was the year Rhoda met Charles. It was in

1850, too, that Philip and Cynthia Derry struck out for Oregon Territory to seek their fortune. Several of the older Derry children were married by 1850 – Basil's first wife Sarah Slater was still alive, Mary Jane was married to Anderson Slater, Sarah's older brother, and Carlisle was married and living in Missouri. The clan must have been thrilled that Rhoda had found love too.

But when that love turned tragic just a couple of years later, maybe the brothers and sisters pulled together in their shared loss. In 1851, Basil lost Sarah and two of their sons. He would remarry in 1852, about the time of Rhoda's confrontation with Nancy Phenix. Philip and Cynthia would both die on their Oregon adventure in 1854, the year Rhoda was admitted to Jacksonville. By 1860, when Rachel died, there had been joys and sorrows aplenty shared between the nine children of Jacob and Rachel Derry.

Did any of Rhoda's brothers or sisters come to visit her one last time at George Jacobs' house before she was taken away to the almshouse? We have no idea. We know her brothers and sisters cared for her very much. The story of Anderson sleeping on a cot next to her bed, to keep her covered on a cold winter night, is testimony to that caring.

We do know Rhoda's story was shared with the family. It was no secret that Rhoda had been put away. Levi Slater, Rhoda's nephew, gave a detailed account of her story to the *Quincy Daily Journal* for an article dated November 23, 1906. Her memory was kept alive for the next generation.

By the time Rhoda was released from the Adams County almshouse in 1904, only one of her siblings was still alive – her brother, James McCann Derry, who was living and farming in Durham, Lewis County, Missouri. But as for who, if anyone, was there to see her committed to the almshouse at the beginning of her ordeal ... well, we just don't know.

It would be comforting, though, to at least imagine Rhoda getting several last hugs from James, or Barbara, or Jerimiah, before she climbed into the wagon that would take her to the almshouse.

It would be comforting – because she would never see her father, or any of her brothers or sisters, again.

The journey to the Adams County almshouse was probably not as dramatic as Rhoda's committal to the state hospital in Jacksonville. Instead of two doctors and the sheriff showing up at the Derry home, it was probably just Jacob hitching up a wagon, packing a bag for Rhoda, and coaxing her onto the seat beside him. Instead of the hundred-mile trip to Jacksonville from Lima, Jacob just had to drive the wagon about twenty-five miles. He probably would have had to drive through Ursa to make his way south, then turn east towards Coatsburg. Did Rhoda feel a flash of pained recognition as the wagon rumbled through Charles' former hometown?

There was less drama on this trip, but no less pain.

Jacob pulled the wagon up in front of the three-story brick building of the Adams County almshouse. He helped Rhoda out of the wagon, and led her through the gate in the white picket fence and into the building. He probably gave her a hug, and a kiss goodbye.

And then he left her there.

We can only guess Rhoda's thoughts at being abandoned like this. Charles had left for parts unknown years before. Her mother, the only person who really understood her fears, who had shot at the invisible witches for her, was gone. Her father had brought her to the almshouse and left her. That first night, the dark slipped in, to crouch in shadow in the corners of the room. Soon, the darkness crept closer, to whisper its cobweb-covered secrets into her ear.

Bereft, abandoned by her family and by everyone she had ever loved, Rhoda began to lash out. She started to cut herself off from the world that had failed her.

The darkest chapter in Rhoda's life was about to begin.

CHAPTER FOURTEEN
HISTORICAL CARE OF THE INSANE

The most famous and infamous of all asylums was Bethlem, London's dumping-ground for the insane. The Priory of St. Mary of Bethlem was founded in 1247 as a way to raise funds for one of the crusading groups, the Order of Bethlehem, The monastery was located on Bishopsgate, and its function was, at first, to take in indigent plague victims, and to collect and distribute alms. Records show that in 1403, there were six madmen at the priory. By 1598, there were twenty, and the monastery was beginning to gain a reputation for treating the insane. In 1650, the number of insane patients had risen to fifty. By then, males and females were separated, and the staff was forbidden to beat the inmates.

Conditions at Bethlem were routinely horrible. The place was filthy – inmates slept on the cold, damp floor, and in 1598, the only water supply was a cistern in the backyard.

The common attitude towards Bethlem asylum in modern times is that it was a freak show, kind of a human zoo where spectators paid for the dubious privilege of gawking at the inmates. Although it is true that paying visitors did stroll through the asylum, modern scholars have decided it wasn't quite as simple or as crass as that. The magnificent architecture of the asylum was the real draw. People donated money – which was used to care for the inmates – to go in and examine the lavish architecture. People didn't actually pay admission; the entrance fee was considered a charitable donation. Bethlem wasn't the only institution to trade spectacle for alms. All kinds of charities – almshouses, hospitals, and orphanages – encouraged philanthropy in return for a tour of the facilities.

Many of the visitors to Bethlem were, in fact, family members who were visiting patients, bearing gifts of extra food, blankets, clothing, even writing material. The supervisors at the asylum encouraged upper-class visitors, feeling that such a clientele would leave tips for the staff and cheer up the patients by their very presence.

In 1770, the supervisors decided to limit visitors more strictly. This was done ostensibly to shield the inmates from curiosity seekers. But it may have been to the inmates' detriment – with visitors apt to pop in any time, the attendants had to at least make a show of caring for the patients. With fewer impromptu guests, the staff grew lax, and were more callous in their treatment of their charges.

SALPETRIERE AND BICETRE

The two major pauper asylums in France were an improvement over London's Bedlam. The hospital at Salpetriere was founded in 1656, and housed in a repurposed saltpeter factory. As a hospital, it served not only the mentally ill, but also patients with venereal disease, the elderly poor, able-bodied but lazy boys, and girls at risk for debauchery.

Philippe Pinel (1745-1826) made his career at these two French asylums. Pinel is considered to be the father of modern psychiatry. A friend of Pinel's committed suicide, and that drove Pinel to pursue a greater understanding of mental illness. He was a passionate reformer, and spent much of his career putting together a workable classification of mental disorders. In 1809, he described a case for the second edition of a textbook on insanity; that case is now regarded as the earliest description of dementia praecox, or schizophrenia, as it became known in the twentieth century.

Pinel's reforms consisted mostly of convincing people that asylums should be places for curing patients, not punishing them. He rejected the use of restraints, preferring instead to talk to the patients in an effort to understand them better. Although later reformers would credit Pinel with "freeing the mad from their chains" it was actually Pinel's assistant, a former mental patient named Poussin, who forbade the use of restraints when he became superintendent of Salpetriere in the 1770s. But more than any other physician, it is Pinel who is now regarded as the one who transformed the concept of "the mad" from deranged lunatics into patients who needed care and understanding.

WILLIAM TUKE AND THE YORK RETREAT

Pinel found great inspiration in the career of William Tuke (1732-1822), a Quaker who lived in York, England. Like Pinel, Tuke had a friend who suffered from mental illness. After the friend died in the York asylum in 1790, Tuke was moved to establish a private asylum for Quakers in York. The York Retreat was founded in 1796. The word "retreat" in the institution's name was chosen to evoke thoughts of a safe haven, a sanctuary from the hustle and bustle of life on the outside. Tuke insisted on a regimen of healthy food, adequate sleep, and good personal hygiene. Like Pinel, he was famous for rejecting the use of mechanical restraints such as shackles and straitjackets.

One of Tuke's novel approaches to patient care was that he offered wholesome, home cooked meals. He noticed that in healthy people, a meal that included cheese and meat – and port – tended to make the diners drowsy. So he included these in the meals he had his staff prepare for his patients. He also encouraged socialization between the patients and his own family members. The whole idea was to make patients feel, literally, at home. Animals, such as rabbits, chickens, and seagulls were to be found on the asylum's grounds, because Tuke felt that interacting with animals would awaken feelings of compassion in his patients.

AMERICAN INSTITUTIONS FOR THE INSANE

Across the pond, Benjamin Franklin and Benjamin Rush established the Pennsylvania Hospital for the care of both mental and medical cases. The hospital accepted people who had "unhappily become disorder'd in their Senses", as Franklin put it, as well as offering medical care. In 1770, the same year that Bethlem forbade people to come in and gawk at the inmates, people in Philadelphia could still peep in the windows of the Pennsylvania Hospital, just as they had been doing for two decades. Passersby would regularly jeer at the insane patients, who were chained, unable to move away from their tormentors.

By 1832, there were 249 patients at the hospital, of which 126 were insane, and housed separately. Harsh medical treatments for insanity were common. Bleeding, purging, and blistering were all used in an attempt to deplete the patient's system.

Even under these appalling circumstances, the Pennsylvania Hospital was just about the best place for the early American lunatic. Most insane people in the colonial period were locked up in jails or almshouses, places that weren't nearly as pleasant as the hospital. Other lunatics lived with their families, dependent on people who were completely untrained in the care of the insane. Or they were just kicked out to wander the countryside.

Conditions in asylums improved during the nineteenth century, though. Care of the insane began to shift towards a theory called "moral management". Treatment of the insane, at least at private asylums, moved from harsh medical practices to a much gentler system. Moral management included talk therapy, occupational therapy for those able to perform light work, and entertainment. Hospitals for the insane now featured billiard tables in the dayrooms and croquet courts on the lawns. Some asylums even offered golf courses, or small wagons so that patients could amuse themselves with a ride.

These little amusements were an essential part of moral management. They were so successful in private asylums that doctors fought for their use at state hospitals too. State legislators, though, didn't always see the reason in this. At the public asylum in Columbia, South Carolina, the builders were forced to eliminate such amusements, as the state lawmakers saw them as frills. The asylum's doctors argued back, saying that occupational therapies and other benefits would attract paying patients, who would offset the cost of treating indigent inmates.

The nineteenth century also saw the rise of the idea of asylum architecture as part of the treatment of the insane. Landscape artists such as Frederick Law Olmsted were invited to design asylum grounds. Landscapes began to include orchards, gardens, and pathways through the grounds, ostensibly for the enjoyment of patients out for a stroll. Even state hospitals, such as the asylum at Jacksonville, benefitted from this design. Landscaping the grounds of an asylum was considered to be just as important as designing the buildings in which the patients were housed. The doctors of the nineteenth century were trying to get as far away from treatments of the eighteenth century as possible. The eighteenth century was the age of chaining patients to walls or locking them in cages. A chained patient wasn't allowed to go outside. Ever. Modern times called for modern methods – including fresh air and nature.

American doctors of the early nineteenth century tended to believe that mental patients were inherently good, and that moral management stood a decent chance of restoring the insane to mental health. To cover all their bases, though, they relied on medical treatment of the insane as well. In addition to talk therapy, recreation, and occupational therapy, doctors prescribed laudanum and other opiates, warm baths, cold baths, and laxatives.

As far as asylum architecture went, no one was more interested in the subject than Dr. Thomas Story Kirkbride. He firmly believed that a new type of building was needed to house the insane, and that the design of that building was essential for curing those patients.

Kirkbride came up with the idea that patients should all be housed together, in one massive building. The idea was that by having all of the inmates together, the superintendent could visit all the male patients daily, while his wife could visit all the female patients, to check on their progress.

Buildings built according to the Kirkbride plan were designed to cure eighty percent of the patients housed there. Good lighting and proper ventilation were essential elements of the building plan. A Kirkbride building featured a large center section, with wings coming off each end in a shallow V construction. This ensured that every ward had good ventilation and an unobstructed view of the grounds.

But even this carefully considered plan had its drawbacks. Nineteenth century doctors felt that the insane really needed to be cared for in an institutionalized setting, rather than at home. They felt that since the patient had developed the mental illness at home, the home setting had contributed to the mania. Removing the patient from that setting was considered the best way to effect a cure. Yet the doctors wanted to put patients in as homey and comfortable an environment as possible. Kirkbride buildings were wonderful – in theory. Patients could look out on the rolling, manicured grounds from any ward in the building. But a Kirkbride building in no way resembled any patient's house. A huge, imposing stone edifice is a far cry from a home. And when the population of an asylum swelled from 250 to 600 patients, as it often did, the superintendent and his wife could no longer manage a daily visit to every patient, despite their best intentions.

Another drawback of the Kirkbride system was that all of the patients were housed together. If you have someone with mild depression sharing a room with a raving schizophrenic, the situation isn't any good for either one of them. The Kirkbride plan was well-meaning, but flawed. The Kirkbride plan's obsolescence became painfully obvious after only a few decades of its use. The shallow V plan of the Kirkbride buildings was so specialized, a linear plan building was very difficult to repurpose into anything but an asylum. Many of the buildings had to be torn down when the asylums closed.

Asylum design soon moved away from the Kirkbride system to the cottage plan. Instead of spending funds on one massive stone building, with all of the heating, cooling, and plumbing headaches that entailed, designers began to build smaller cottages and wards using wood and brick. Heating and plumbing several smaller buildings was a much more economical choice.

PRIVATE HOSPITALS, STATE HOSPITALS, AND ALMSHOUSES

Until Dorothea Dix started campaigning for state hospitals in the 1840s, all of this dickering over the proper way to build an asylum only benefitted those patients who could pay to be there. Anyone could be affected by mental illness – that hasn't changed between then and now. Insanity cut its swathe across all levels of society, just as it does today. Some patients could afford private asylums, and some had to settle for state hospitals.

There was a wide range in spending between private and public asylums. In 1872, the average weekly expenditure per patient at private asylums was $10.33, while state hospitals spent an average of $4.33 per patient. (Superintendents at state hospitals argued, though, that their economy didn't affect the basic comforts offered to patients.)

Superintendents at private asylums pointed out that since their affluent patients were accustomed to having privacy and luxury in health, it made sense to allow them to enjoy the same accommodations while in the asylum. Being surrounded with the comforts of home, especially if those comforts were opulent, would help the patient recover faster. And some wealthy families chose private asylums for their loved ones so that their ailing relatives wouldn't have to mix with inmates of a lower social class.

Sometimes, though, private hospitals accepted a small number of impoverished patients. Most poor New Yorkers, for example, had to seek treatment for insanity at Blackwell's Island asylum, which was run by the city (and where conditions were ghastly). But the privately-run Bloomingdale Asylum, an exclusive hospital for the wealthy, was obligated to take in a small percentage of poor folks because part of its funding came from the state. Even so, treatment was offered only to "indigent persons of superior respectability" – clergymen and teachers, mostly.

This isn't to say private asylums were places of serene perfection, though. A patient who had voluntarily committed herself to Bloomingdale wrote in 1872 that conditions were not as rosy as patients' families were led to believe. She wrote that the shower-bath was used as an instrument of torture, that whenever a patient complained, the doctors always believed the attendants' version of events, rather than what the patients reported, and that the food was "more suitable ... for dogs and cats than human beings". Abuse could happen in private asylums just the same as in public hospitals.

The idea of state hospitals had been discussed as early as 1838. It was the ceaseless campaigning of Dorothea Dix that jumpstarted the whole process. Before Dix started her crusade, many indigent insane were suffering in prisons or almshouses. Dix made it her mission to bring legislators' attention to the dire plight of the impoverished mentally ill. Those who couldn't afford care in a private hospital often ended up in prison. County officials, lacking anywhere else to send them, placed the insane poor in county almshouses when they were a danger to themselves and others.

Dix made an economic argument for building state hospitals. Many doctors believed mental illness could be cured. Therefore, Dix argued, it would cost the state less to support a patient for the short time they would spend in a hospital, than it would to pay for them to spend the rest of their life in the poorhouse.

Almshouses, or poorhouses, were strictly no-frills affairs. They were intended to give poor folks a place to live – they were in no way designed to help the insane recover from mental illness. There were no doctors in residence at almshouses – the doctor came in every so often to attend to the physical complaints of the residents, usually at his own cost. The usual arrangement of an almshouse was to keep the paupers in a large building, with a "backhouse" hidden away for housing the insane residents.

In the worst cases, anyone with $25 for the license and an unused barn in their backyard could, in theory, open and run an almshouse. Many indigent insane ended up in situations like this, because laypeople didn't think the insane could feel heat, or cold, or hunger. In the *very* worst cases, the mentally ill were treated no better than animals.

This is what led Dorothea Dix to fight so hard for state hospitals. She realized the importance of having a place to treat the impoverished insane that had more oversight than the almshouses. State hospitals provided a safe place for the mentally ill to seek treatment, even if they couldn't afford the luxury of a private asylum. The accommodations weren't as fancy as the wards of private asylums. But even state hospitals had well-landscaped grounds, decent food, and shelter.

A look at almshouses in Illinois in 1881 reveals a lot about conditions all over the state. It's an intriguing mix of good and bad – superintendents trying to do the best they could, and inmates, particularly the insane, living in unimaginable squalor.

In Kane County, the poorhouse held 425 paupers, of whom fifteen were insane. Of those, two were in seclusion, but none were in restraint. "The keeper objects to the statement made in the last report of the board of charities that the county has never treated its insane well. This remark is based partly upon the fact that one of its insane has been kept in chains for many years, except when in seclusion. The keeper states that the man is so violent that it is absolutely dangerous to enter his cell, and that he (the keeper) has often been knocked down by him ... such a patient should not be kept upon the county farm at all, but sent to the state hospital at Elgin..."

Effingham County didn't have a poorhouse. Instead, paupers were housed in the old courthouse at Ewington. In 1881, there were seventeen inmates, five of whom were insane. "This [building] is so dilapidated that it would fall to pieces if it were not tied together by iron rods crossing in every direction. The furniture is poor in quality and meagre [sic] in quantity. The bedding is dirty, worn out, and some of it almost rotten. The county does not furnish bedding, and the result is that each new contractor buys of his predecessor the bedding already on hand, which accounts for its shameful condition."

Conditions were even worse in Gallatin County. Again, there was no poorhouse for the county. Rather, the county "leased" its paupers to a single contractor, who furnished food, clothing, medicine, and the doctor's visits, in return for $1.80 per week for every pauper (paid by the county). The buildings in which these people lived were shanties, not plastered on the inside, with cracks between the boards; they were in no way weather proof, or even fit for human habitation. The report noted that the inmates were all very poorly clad. "A little girl, about seven years of age, was going around barefoot, who had not had on a shoe or stocking for over a year."

In Lake County, there were thirty-seven inmates, twelve of whom were insane (nine women, three men). "It is rather remarkable, that the county fairground is upon the county farm, and visitors to the fair appear to regard the 'crazy house', as it is called, as the greatest attraction of the occasion. A German boy, who resides in the neighborhood, was so upset by an insane woman spitting at him through the grated door as to require medical care, at times, for three or four years afterward."

The squalor was just as bad in LaSalle County, where 108 inmates lived. There were sixty-one insane there – twenty-two men, thirty-nine women. "The condition of the building for the care of the insane is horrible. The impression upon a spectator is inexpressibly disgusting. Six of them, most of whom are entirely naked, are confined in an out-house, where they lie upon the floor in their own filth, without care or attention other than that which an aged pauper is able to give them. Their appearance reminds one of hogs upon the floor of a pig-sty. At the time of our former visit, two years ago, the officer representing this board was prevented from going to this house by the county agent, who falsely informed him that all the insane inmates had been seen by him. Since that time the agent has been changed."

The tone of the report for Rock Island (ninety-three inmates – thirty-six insane, being twenty men and sixteen women) is one of weary impatience. "We fully described this almshouse two years ago, and there has been no improvement since. The establishment is overcrowded, badly arranged and badly managed. The discipline is not good – and there is little, if anything, about the place which deserves commendation. The insane department is a nuisance, and should be abated." The report makes special note of one of the inmates, although it does not mention if he is one of the insane, or simply poor. "One inmate of this establishment, a man about thirty years of age, cannot walk erect, but travels on all-fours [sic], and succeeds in making very good time. What is strange to report, he is said to be quite an expert player upon the violin, but he cannot dance to his own music."

Fortunately, not all poorhouses were such abysmal holes. The Fulton County almshouse was the home of forty-eight inmates. "In our last report respecting Fulton County, we said: 'This farm occupies a beautiful site; the main building is good; the inmates are well fed and tolerably well clothed; but there is a general lack of neatness and cleanliness, both in the premises and in the paupers themselves, which has been noticeable at every visit made by us for ten years. The filth around the house is offensive; the portion of the house occupied by the male paupers has a bad smell; and the insane department is so neglected that it is one of the most forlorn in the state; the cells are very dirty.' We are happy to say that a new keeper has been appointed, who took charge in October, 1879, and there is a marked improvement in the condition of the almshouse, in every respect ... the rooms are clean, and a pure atmosphere pervades the whole institution."

In Henry County, where the almshouse cared for forty-eight inmates, eight of whom were insane, the mentally ill weren't treated too badly. "None of the insane are in seclusion, or in any way restrained of their liberty, and their condition is one of personal comfort. Two of them are said to be capable of farm labor, and two of labor about the house."

Jo Daviess County, with forty-six inmates, seven of whom were insane, had a very long way to go, but the county was working on improving the lot of the insane. Here, the mentally ill were always kept in cells, and let out only when the cells were being cleaned. "This constant seclusion is undoubtedly a great wrong to the helpless victims", the report reads with a note of sorrow. The report does say that the county was in the process of building a new home just for the purpose of housing its insane poor.

The insane of Morgan County (sixty inmates, twenty-eight insane) were cared for very well. "The rooms in which the insane are kept are clean and well ventilated, and the bedding [is] clean and comfortable. This department is a model of neatness; no dirt is perceptible, even in the cells of those who are most uncleanly in their habits. The inmates are kindly treated, and prompt attention is given to all their wants."

It's interesting to ask, at this point, if the superintendent's salary had anything to do with the care the poor received. Louis Fredlander, who had been the superintendent of the Morgan County almshouse since 1871, got a salary from the county board of $900, and his wife got $300 for helping him. The superintendent for LaSalle County's almshouse, which was wretched, got only $800.

Ira Pendley, in charge of the paupers housed in the old courthouse in Effingham County, got just $1.16 per week for every inmate – but with seventeen inmates, that worked out to $1025.44 in 1880. And in Rock Island County, home of the crippled violin player, the report noted that "the keeper has been in charge since 1861, and is paid $1000 a year for his services but is tired of the position". Apparently, wages on the high end of the scale were no protection against job burnout.

The best place to be a poor person (at least in 1881) was in Knox County. The poorhouse there was home to 105 inmates, of whom twenty-eight were insane (thirteen men, fifteen women, none in seclusion or restraint). "This almshouse is supplied with all the modern improvements, and all the rooms are well if not elegantly furnished. Carpets are found on the floors of nearly all the rooms, and the walls are generally adorned with pictures. The establishment is first-class in every respect, and great credit is due Mrs. Cleaveland, the superintendent, who rules thoroughly, while not seeming to rule at all. She has held her position since the year 1867, and is paid a salary of $800."

"In our last report, mention was made of one female patient who occupies a large wooden box filled with straw. She will not wear clothing, but is covered with a canvass cloth, is in constant motion, has bruised herself from head to foot, and put out her own eyes. This patient is still an occupant of the box referred to..."

The *Reports Made to the General Assembly of Illinois* for 1881 begins with Adams County. (Alphabetical order suits a bureaucracy.) The report notes that the county owned a farm as well as a poorhouse. The superintendent, who in 1881 was William Elliott, was paid $40 a month – only $480 a year – but the county board paid all of the expenses incurred in maintaining the almshouse.

At the time of the report, there were a hundred and one paupers living at the Adams County almshouse. The report noted that "the rooms and bedding were found to be clean and in good condition, and the inmates appeared to be in good health and well cared for". In short, there really wasn't anything to set the Adams County almshouse apart from any of the other county poorhouses in Illinois.

Except for the woman in the box.

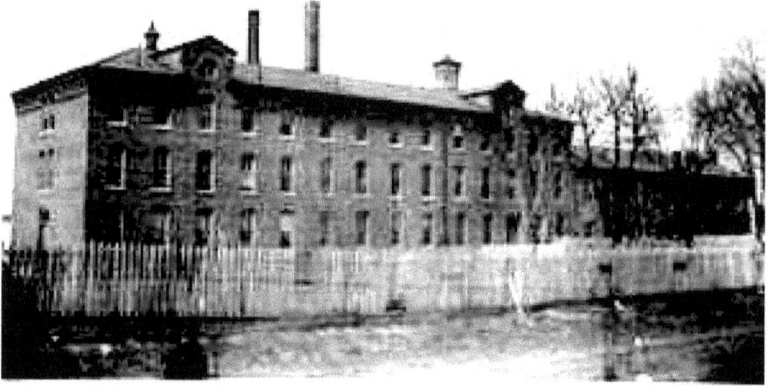

CHAPTER FIFTEEN
THE ADAMS COUNTY ALMSHOUSE

Illinois became a state in 1818. Public care of the poor began the very next year.

At first, the destitute of the state were cared for by private citizens appointed by public officials. This "farm out" system meant that the poor, who were being given assistance by other settlers, became objects of charity. Even though they were physically able to work, there were no jobs available for them, and they were not financially stable enough to buy their own land to farm.

Within twenty years, this farm out system was replaced by the county poorhouse. By 1839, counties were authorized to establish poorhouses, to hire keepers to oversee these homes, and to levy a property tax for poorhouse support. These institutions took in not only the destitute, but also those suffering from "bodily infirmity (or) idiocy". (By 1919, attitudes towards the poor had changed. Being poor was no longer seen as a sin or moral failing. Contemptuous terms like poorhouse, almshouse, and poor farm were replaced with the more neutral "county home".)

In 1847, the same year that the Illinois Hospital for the Insane was founded in Jacksonville, Adams County purchased the eighty-acre farm of H. T. Ellis in Honey Creek Township for use as a poor farm. The county spent $700 on March 16, 1847, to purchase the land, along with the two story frame house, the barn, the blacksmith shop, and other outbuildings that stood on the property. The poor of the county began to trickle in. Anyone who arrived, male or female, was issued some light work. This poorhouse was in service until May, 1855.

For the first three years, the paupers were under the charge of one man, who received a weekly stipend for their care. Later, the county Board of Supervisors decided to manage the almshouse themselves. They appointed a superintendent for the day-to-day running of the institution.

The Board of Supervisors for the Adams County almshouse met in January 1856, and appointed a committee to find a larger farm and arrange for more buildings for the care of the county's charges. By June of that year, the committee purchased a much larger piece of property from John F. Battell, a 160-acre farm in the northeast quarter of Gilmer Township. The committee spent $5,000 on the new property, and bought fifty thousand bricks with which to start building the new poorhouse.

The building was ready by the next year, and in 1857, the Adams County almshouse opened its doors to the destitute. Fifteen people moved from the old farm to the new property. By 1860, the population had increased to twenty-five – including Rhoda Derry. In 1863, the county built an addition to the first building. Like the original, the new home was two stories high, with a basement.

In 1862, when Rhoda had been at the almshouse for two years, the county built a home specifically for the insane, at a cost of $1,000. One of the superintendents, David L. Hair, wrote that the building was later taken down, "since it did not give satisfaction as a place to confine the insane". The mentally ill returned to the main building, and rejoined the general population.

By 1874, county poorhouse records were required to note admission, discharge, place of birth, cause of dependence on the poorhouse, and other vital information. The Adams County almshouse registers show name, sex, age, color, birthplace, occupation before admission, marital status and former residence of the inmate, the birthplace of the inmate's parents, health status, personal habits (as far as being abstinent, temperate, or a drunkard), a list of property brought to the almshouse, the dates of admission and discharge, and, if the inmate died while staying at the almshouse, the date of death. The register also showed whether the inmate's dependence on the county's generosity resulted from idiocy, lunacy, intemperance, or other causes.

In 1874, the city of Quincy reorganized its care of paupers. The poor of Quincy were transferred to the Adams County almshouse as well. This influx of people overwhelmed the institution, so the County Board arranged a temporary partnership with the Charitable Aid and Hospital Association of Quincy. This arrangement lasted from July 1, 1874 to April 30, 1876.

With this coming surge in population, the Board recommended that a new building be built to house the indigent of Adams County. They suggested a building three stories high, and appropriated $8,000 for its construction. (It came in under budget, being finished in 1875 at a cost of $7,968.) The steam heating system and other modern touches, installed afterward, added another $2,000 to the tab.

Construction continued. By 1897, the almshouse needed somewhere to house its insane inmates, including Rhoda. The county ponied up $10,000 for a new building specifically for their charges who were mentally ill. It was only slightly smaller than the main building. Then came various outbuildings, a new heating plant, and other improvements, as the population of the poorhouse continued to grow.

So far, so good. For the indigent citizens of Quincy and Adams County, the poorhouse was not a horrible place to be. Able-bodied folks who showed up there were given light work to do, in exchange for three hots and a cot. They got to see a doctor if they needed one. The poor farm provided a necessary social service, in a pleasantly bucolic setting.

But the Adams County almshouse was not equipped to care for the mentally ill. Reports of substandard conditions for the insane inmates showed up in local newspapers every so often. An article in the *Quincy Daily Journal*, dated February 12, 1892, pointed to neglect and a certain amount of abuse at the poor farm. The article mentioned that "a simple-minded woman had charge of the insane women's department, food distribution etc." A later report stated that there were only two women – a matron and an "insane servant" – available to care for ninety-four residents.

The Adams County almshouse had its share of problems. But it was located in 160 acres of lovely farmland, including a newly-built home for the poor, another brand-new home for the insane and feeble-minded, several outbuildings sufficient for the farm's needs, and five acres of orchard. David L. Hair, one of the previous superintendents of the Adams County Poor Farm, wrote in *Past and*

Present of Adams County, that "it is said that there is not a better managed poor farm in the state, for the management has always been good. The poor are liberally provided for, and at the same time the management has been so economical that the County Poor Farm is a credit to the Adams County tax payers."

The staff of the farm made sure that those indigent who came to them for help that wanted to work for their keep could do so. Those that couldn't, the infirm or the insane, were cared for as well – maybe not in optimum circumstances, but they were cared for nonetheless. This was not the homestead of one of the unscrupulous farmers who opened their drafty barn to take in the mentally ill. This was an institution built specifically for the care of the indigent of Adams County – that also happened to get saddled with the destitute mentally ill who could not afford to go to the state hospital at Jacksonville, or who had been deemed by the doctors at Jacksonville to be incurable.

And what about the men in charge of the Adams County poor farm? During the time that Rhoda Derry lived there, there were seven men – and one woman – who held the position of superintendent of the Adams County almshouse. (Mrs. Doren took over the position after her husband died, and held it for six years.) We do have "biographical sketches" of a couple of these men – William Bates and Jacob Wolfe. Bates was superintendent from 1889 to 1895. Wolfe was superintendent from 1901 to 1905 – he would have been in charge in September 1904, when Dr. Zeller made his fateful visit to Adams County. Let's meet these men, and see if they are indeed the ogres who locked Rhoda in a Utica crib for decades on end.

William I. Bates was born in Tennessee in 1828, a son of Joseph and Nancy B. Bates. When grown, he farmed 160 acres in Hancock County Illinois for twenty years. After that, he moved to Chicago to try his hand at the livestock business. That didn't seem to work as well, for he soon sold out. He moved back down south to Adams County, and again farmed for ten years. It was at that point that Bates was appointed superintendent of the Adams County poor farm.

So what kind of superintendent was he? He started around 1889, and served in the position for six years. The *Portrait and Biographical Record of Adams County, Illinois* has this to say about William Bates:

> "In early life, Mr. Bates was a supporter of the Democratic party, but on account of his strong temperance principles, is Prohibitionist in sentiment. Socially, he is a Knight Templar Mason and himself, wife, and children are all members of the

Methodist Episcopal Church, to the support of which he contributes liberally. The poor and needy have ever found in him a friend. He is charitable and benevolent, generous, warm-hearted and true. His life is well worthy of emulation, and by his upright, honorable career he has won many warm friends."

(It's interesting to note that the Methodist Episcopal Church is mentioned as having a presence in Ursa, Charles Phenix's home town, too. It was a thriving part of frontier society in that part of Illinois.)

It looks like William Bates was not in charge for the growth spurts of the poor farm. (It was two years after he stepped down, in 1897, that the new home for the insane was built.) But he seems to have been a capable, well-liked member of his church and his community.

How about Jacob B. Wolfe, the superintendent of the poor farm who was overseeing things when Dr. Zeller arrived in 1904 to rescue Rhoda? We can find information on his life in the book *Quincy and Adams County History and Representative Men* (Volume 2).

Jacob Wolfe was born in Liberty Township in Illinois on April 9, 1850, to Elder David and Pamela Ann (Francis) Wolfe. Elder David Wolfe, Jacob's father, helped establish the Dunkard Church in Liberty. There were several preachers in the congregation, but only one elder. Elder Wolfe's jurisdiction included Adams, Pike, and Hancock counties. His work as a missionary took him all over the counties, and many times, to Indiana. On occasion, he preached as far away as Texas.

Jacob seems to have inherited his father's sense of duty, but he channeled it into politics and civil service, rather than religion.

"Jacob B. Wolfe was well educated in Liberty and also attended the Quincy Business College. He lived in Liberty Township forty years, and most of that time owned and operated his grandfather's old farm. About 1898 he moved to Quincy as deputy sheriff under John W. Roth, serving as turnkey in charge of the prisoners at the county jail. For about fifteen years he served as a member of the County Board of Supervisors, representing Liberty Township, and was finally selected by the Board as superintendent of the County Poor Farm. His administration was a most capable as well as a most kindly and effective one. During his term the number of inmates at the farm was 100, though at times the number rose as high as 180. He was occupied with the responsibilities of this institution for four years ... He is one of the best known men in the county. He has long been active in the Democratic party, serving as county committee man in Liberty Township, and is in every sense a public spirited citizen. He was reared in the old family church at Liberty, but has had no active part in it for many years. For over thirty years he has been affiliated with the Liberty Lodge of Masons, has held all the chairs and for three years sat on the Grand Lodge. He is one of the oldest members of the Liberty Lodge."

The character of these men just deepens Rhoda's mystery. The superintendents at the Adams County almshouse were not bad guys. They were churchgoers, devout Christians, responsible citizens, pillars of their community. At least two of them were respected Masons. Jacob Wolfe had "held all the chairs" – meaning he had volunteered for every position that needed to be filled in a Masonic lodge. They were not cruel, heartless monsters. They were men who stepped up and took on the responsibility of caring for the poor, the indigent, the destitute – and yes, some of the insane of Adams County.

So how in the world did Rhoda Derry end up spending forty-four years locked in a cage?

The answer lies in the times in which these people lived. Simply being poor wasn't seen as a sin, or even a fault. The well-off citizens of Illinois realized they had to shoulder the burden of caring for people who weren't so fortunate, and this they did. They began by opening their homes. Later, the counties established dedicated poor farms.

The mentally ill, on the other hand, were a different story. Then, as now, there was a stigma attached to mental illness, harder to shake than a prairie burr in a horse's mane. The insane *were* blamed for their condition. The mentally ill were considered subhuman. This led to the abuses seen under the old system, where anyone with $25 for the license fee and an empty barn could open an almshouse for the insane. They were treated, in some cases, no better than animals. There was no oversight, no therapy, no care as there was in a state hospital. There was no separation of the sexes – insane women were often sexually abused by the male inmates. (In the early days of the Peoria State Hospital, when Dr. Zeller was opening the doors of the asylum to the insane population of Illinois' almshouses, many women came to the asylum pregnant.)

These conditions led to a haughty, impatient attitude towards the mentally ill who were also poor. No matter their affliction – depression, epilepsy, dementia – they were lumped together as "insane", or "lunatics". (Those with developmental disabilities were labelled "idiots", or "feeble-minded".) The indigent mentally ill weren't even given the luxury of the care they would have received at the state hospital in Jacksonville. There were no conversations with doctors, no therapeutic strolls on the manicured grounds, no soothing doses of laudanum.

The developmentally disabled had the most difficulty – there was absolutely no place for them outside their own family circle. If they were turned out of their homes, or lost their family somehow, they were out of luck. The state hospital wasn't equipped to care for the mentally handicapped. The feeble-minded living on their own were doomed to almshouses.

This all led to a mindset of "this is why we can't have nice things" on the part of the people in charge of the county poorhouses. The superintendents and staff of the county farms took in the poor and gave them work to do. The insane, though, were either incapable of work, or able to do only the most basic of chores. Through no fault of their own, they were seen as burdens rather than as charity cases. Almshouses were designed to give the poor a helping hand – they were not designed for the care of the mentally ill.

And Rhoda Derry would have been a handful for any institution that took her in. Even if she'd been able to go back to Jacksonville, she'd have been put right back into the ward for deeply troubled patients. No one connected with the poor farm – not David Hair, the superintendent in charge in 1860, when Rhoda arrived, not the Board of Supervisors, not the feeble-minded servant, *no one* – was prepared to deal with Rhoda's depth of crazy.

At that point in her life, Rhoda had lost everything. She had lost Charles. She had lost her mother. She had lost her family. The sense of betrayal and abandonment she felt must have been profound. In the depths of her despair, she began to act out.

Rhoda was a very violent patient. Her clothes had to be tied on her – otherwise she would just rip them off in her rages.

Tying her clothes on was also the staff's solution to another habit of Rhoda's – she developed pica in the almshouse. Pica is a disorder in which a sufferer tries to eat inappropriate objects. It began with Rhoda picking the buttons off of her blouse and swallowing them. (Hence the need to tie her now-buttonless blouse shut.) Then she would lunge at the staff and other inmates, trying to snatch the buttons from their clothes as well.

The random things Rhoda shoved into her mouth were not limited to relatively harmless buttons. Chicken bones were crunched without a second thought. She would also cram things she found on the floor into her mouth – sharp things. Anything Rhoda found – pennies, pins, slivers of wood – she tried to eat.

This habit may have led to the loss of her ability to speak. Famously, when Rhoda arrived at the Peoria State Hospital, she never spoke, but only jabbered. Only some of this was because of her having beaten her front teeth in. It's possible that Rhoda put something sharp into her mouth that lacerated her tongue. She certainly wasn't brushing her teeth at that point, and whatever she put into her mouth (probably from the floor) was crawling with germs. This may have led to gangrene. Her tongue may have been so damaged that she lost the power of speech. As gruesome as this scenario is, it may be a possible explanation for her inability to speak, even after she reached the safe haven of the Peoria State Hospital.

The superintendent of the almshouse, David Hair, gave the order to lock Rhoda in a Utica crib, for her own safety.

CHAPTER SIXTEEN
A "HUMANE" APPARATUS

In January 1843, the first patients were admitted to the New York State Lunatic Asylum in Utica, New York, later known as the Utica State Hospital. This was New York State's first publicly funded institution for the treatment of the mentally ill. Under the direction of Dr. Avariah Brigham, the first superintendent, the asylum at Utica thrived. The institution began publishing the *American Journal of Insanity* the next year, in 1844. The publication, the first psychiatric journal in English, soon cemented the asylum's reputation world-wide as a center of psychiatry. (The publication later became known as the *American Psychiatric Journal*, and is still published today.)

Dr. Brigham found existing types of patient restraints unacceptable. In his search for an aid to patient care, he came across a contraption that had been designed in France in 1845, by Dr. M. H. Aubanel of the Marseilles Lunatic Asylum. It was an adult-sized bed that was completely enclosed on all four sides, with a lockable lid on top that was attached with hinges. The lid and sides were made of spindles, which allowed for air flow. The bottom of the crib was made of woven wire, and lined with a thick hospital mattress. The crib was built to the measurements of an average adult – eighteen inches deep, six feet long, and three feet wide.

Dr. Brigham adopted the French design and brought it to the forefront of modern psychiatric care. The Utica State Hospital was one of the first institutions in the United States to use the bed, beginning in 1846. As a result, the bed quickly became known in popular parlance as the "Utica crib".

The Utica crib was a standard piece of equipment in many asylums for about thirty years. Patients actually asked to use it. It gave some patients a sense of safe enclosure, of security, of being tucked away from the world. One patient, prone to sleepwalking, preferred to sleep in the crib. He said if he went to sleep locked in the crib, he knew exactly where he was going to wake up.

Many professionals supported its use, too. In the February 1878 issue of the *Edinburgh Medical Journal*, a Dr. Lindsay and other physicians at the Murray Royal Institution at Perth recommended the Utica crib, saying that it was practical

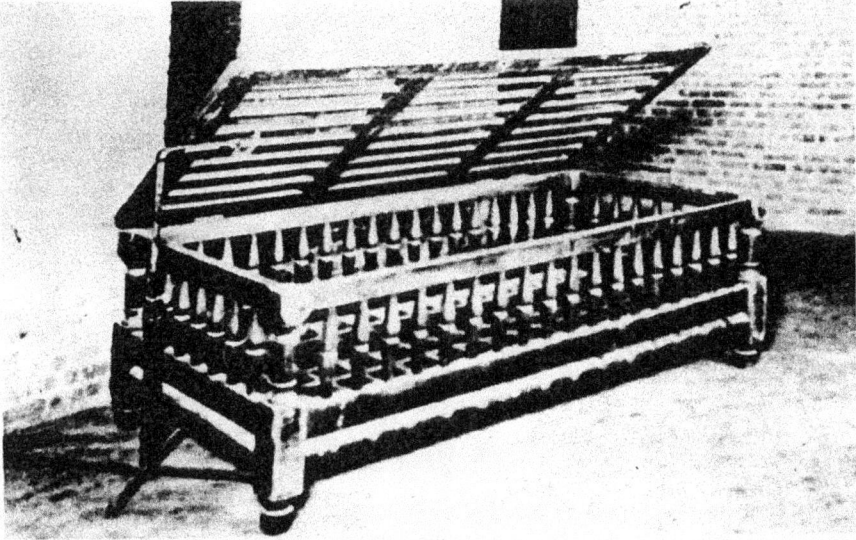

and safe for patients. And the British psychology expert Daniel Tuke specifically mentioned "the celebrated Utica asylum, where a suicidal woman was preserved from harm by this enclosure". A reporter from the *New York Herald* tried out a Utica crib, and pronounced it quite comfortable. He was satisfied with his ability to stretch out and turn over with ease, even to lift his head to look down at his feet while locked in the crib.

Even Dr. George Zeller, with his loathing of restraint of any kind, weighed in on the Utica crib. In his autobiography, he seemed to consider it, if not ideal, at least better than a straitjacket.

"The Utica crib is nothing more than a bed with strong and high wood sides and ends and a swinging door over the top. In it the patient has perfect bodily freedom, limited only by the dimensions of the enclosure. Let anyone witness the writhing and contortions of a patient in a restraint sheet tied hand and foot in bed, or study the interference of respiration while wearing the straight jacket or camisole with arms crossed over the breast and the hands tied across the back by means of the blind sleeve, and see if he would not prefer even the monstrosity known as the Utica crib."

But the Utica crib had its detractors too. Dr. William A. Hammond and Dr. Mycert of the Utica State Hospital – the institution which gave the Utica crib its name – attacked the use of the crib, comparing it to a coffin. In an interview with that same New York Herald reporter, Dr. Hammond admitted that patients had died from being confined in the crib. Many died from panic and shock. Other patients died because attendants forced them into the crib thinking they were out of control, when in reality, they were experiencing a heart attack, stroke, or other acute medical emergency. Eventually, the Utica crib fell from favor, and its use was discontinued. On January 18, 1887, Dr. George Alder Blumer, the third superintendent of the Utica State Hospital, ordered all Utica cribs removed from the asylum.

Whatever its uses, abuses, benefits, or flaws, the Utica crib was never designed for use any longer than overnight. The fact that Rhoda Derry was confined in a crib for days and weeks on end is appalling. She was kept in there constantly. Whoever made the decision to keep her caged up made some adjustments to the crib's design: instead of being lined with a hospital mattress, Rhoda's crib was lined with straw, with a hole cut at a strategic place in the wooden bottom. There was also a tray underneath the hole, to catch the waste.

Rhoda's hips atrophied from her lack of exercise. When she was let out, she could no longer stand upright – she was reduced to crawling along the floor on her hands and knees. On the few occasions when she was let out, she was cared for by other feeble-minded patients.

It is impossible to overstate the misery Rhoda knew in the Adams County Almshouse. Most of us wouldn't last a week locked up in a cage. But Rhoda spent years of her life locked away. She lay there, alone with her thoughts, as the days bled into one another. She lay there, still aching with missing Charles, her mind on fire with madness. It's no wonder she clawed her own eyes out sometime in those first ten years. It was just one less sense to dull over time. Maybe she thought it was better to lose the sense of sight all at once, than watch the world go by from between the bars of a Utica crib.

CHAPTER SEVENTEEN
TIME SLIPS AWAY — 1860-1904

Forty-four years is a long time – a generation, maybe even two. A lot can happen in forty-four years. And a lot *did* happen. The whole time that Rhoda lay in her Utica crib, twitching, jerking, muttering, the years passed.

Rhoda was committed to the Adams County Almshouse on September 3, 1860. Just over two months later, on November 6, 1860, Abraham Lincoln was elected president, and the country lurched a step closer to civil war. The whole horrible bloody business – Fort Sumter, Bull Run, Shiloh, Sherman's March to the Sea, the immortal words spoken at Gettysburg, Antietam, Appomattox, Ford's Theater – took up just a small part of Rhoda's stay in the almshouse.

Lincoln was elected president the year Rhoda was committed. He took the job over from James Buchanan. Five years later, Lincoln was dead. Lincoln was followed by Andrew Johnson, who was followed by Ulysses S. Grant. Then came Rutherford B. Hayes, then James Garfield. After Garfield was felled by Charles Guiteau's bullet only four months into his presidency, Chester A. Arthur took over. Grover Cleveland came next, then Benjamin Harrison, then Cleveland (again). William McKinley declared war on Spain, and Theodore Roosevelt led his Rough Riders up San Juan Hill in Cuba. Later, Teddy Roosevelt took over the reins of the presidency. In all, eleven men sat as president – one of them twice – while Rhoda tossed and turned on her bed of straw.

Laura Ingalls Wilder was born in 1867. Her sister Mary lost her sight in 1879, when Laura was twelve. Rhoda had been in the almshouse for nineteen years. (She lost her sight earlier than Mary Ingalls did; Rhoda clawed her eyes out sometime in her first ten years in the almshouse.) Laura Ingalls married Almanzo Wilder in 1885, when she was eighteen. Their daughter, Rose, was born the next year.

In early October 1871, fires broke out in the hot, dry Great Lakes area. The Great Chicago Fire started October 8. It burned itself out two days later, on Rhoda's thirty-seventh birthday. The Great Chicago Fire killed some three hundred people, and left more than 100,000 residents homeless. On the same day the fire started in Chicago, a firestorm raged through Peshtigo, Wisconsin, 240 miles north of the Windy City. The Peshtigo fire incinerated the town and the surrounding countryside with superheated flames of at least 2000 degrees Fahrenheit. In terms of lives lost, the Peshtigo Fire is the worst natural disaster in American history. The fire killed around fifteen hundred people, and possibly as many as twenty-five hundred.

Scott Joplin was born in 1868. He started his first band in order to perform at the World's Fair in Chicago in 1893. (He played cornet.) The 1893 Columbian Exposition popularized ragtime, and Joplin was off to a great start. He published the "Maple Leaf Rag" in 1899, and "The Entertainer" in 1902.

In 1879, Thomas Edison invented the light bulb. Rhoda never saw the glow of electric lighting. She had been blind for at least ten years, maybe more.

In 1887, Nellie Bly, the investigative reporter, talked her way into the offices of the *New York World*, the newspaper owned by Joseph Pulitzer. She had a daring plan ~ to get herself checked in to Bellevue Hospital, then committed to Blackwell's Island in New York. Later, she wrote the expose` *Ten Days in a Mad House.* Her account of asylum life included descriptions of dangerous patients tied together with ropes, and rats running freely around the hospital. Baths were nothing but buckets of cold water sloshed over the patients. The food consisted of gruel broth, spoiled beef, bread that was little more than dried-out dough, and dirty water. After Bly's release, a grand jury investigated the conditions at Blackwell's Island. The investigation eventually led to a call for increased funding for the care of the insane. The budget of the Department of Public Charities and Corrections was increased by $850,000, and future examinations were made more stringent, so that the only patients admitted to the asylum were those who were truly insane. In 1894, Blackwell's Island was declared unfit for human habitation, and was closed down.

In 1889, Jane Addams founded Hull House, to help the destitute immigrant population of Chicago.

In 1899, Al Capone was born in New York City.

Between 1860 and 1904, the number of stars on our flag went from thirty-three to forty-five.

And through it all, throughout the days and months and years, Rhoda lay in her crib. The mice ran over her wasted limbs and sniffed at the empty sockets where her eyes had been. She lay there, huddled, twitching, betrayed by her body, her mind, her heart.

Until the day in September when everything changed.

PART THREE: THE RESCUE

CHAPTER EIGHTEEN
DR. GEORGE A. ZELLER

When George Zeller was a young boy, he loved to go swimming in the Illinois River. He wrote in his autobiography that on a hot summer's day, when the call "Let's go swimming!" came, it would take him mere moments to strip down and plunge into the cool dark waters.

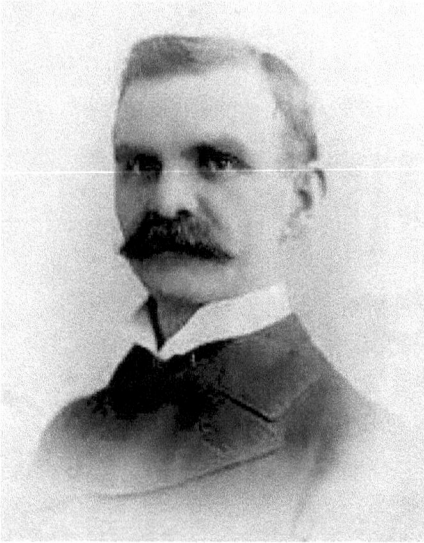

One day, though, that innocent childhood fun turned tragic. A friend of George's splashed happily into the river to swim. Something went wrong – there was a struggle for air, a gulp of river water instead – and the boy was pulled lifeless from the water. George stood by and watched helplessly as his friend died. Later, George would know resuscitation techniques. But as a child, he knew nothing that would help.

That childhood tragedy propelled George Zeller into a life of service, along the path of medicine. Dr. Zeller was born in 1858 in Spring Bay, Illinois, about ten miles north of Peoria on the east bank of the Illinois River. His father, Dr. John George Zeller, came to America from Germany in 1846, at the age of eighteen. He spent two years travelling, then returned to Germany. Unrest in his native country forced him out four years after that, and the elder Dr. Zeller returned to America. He attended medical school at the University of St. Louis, Missouri, then settled in Spring Bay.

Dr. John Zeller passed down to his son "a fierce love of liberty, a strict sense of duty, hatred of oppression, and utter respect for the dignity of man," according to a short biography written by Dr. Zeller's colleague Dr. Maxim Pollak. From his mother, George Zeller inherited "a tender heart, shrinking from abuse in any form".

George Zeller wasn't a stellar student in his early years, but he pulled it together to go to medical school. He attended the University of Illinois for three years, then moved to the Medical Department of the University of St. Louis, following in his father's footsteps. He graduated in March 1879, and came home to go into practice with his father, who was still a well-respected physician in Spring Bay. In 1889, he married Sophie Kline. (Lorado Taft, the celebrated sculptor of such works as the Black Hawk statue in Oregon, Illinois, and *Eternal Silence* at Graceland Cemetery in Chicago, and a classmate of Zeller's at the University of Illinois, was best man at the fashionable wedding.) George and Sophie honeymooned for six months in Europe, where George visited clinics in Berlin and London and attended lectures by Joseph Lister, among others. When they returned to America, they settled in Peoria, where Dr. Zeller established a lucrative practice.

Since childhood, Dr. Zeller had been a great admirer of Abraham Lincoln, and in adulthood he became a staunch Republican. He was instrumental in helping Governor Tanner get elected. In return, Tanner offered Zeller the position of superintendent at the new asylum being planned just outside Peoria, in Bartonville. Bored with the drudgery of day-to-day practice, Zeller accepted the post.

The asylum was still under construction, so in a burst of patriotism, Dr. Zeller volunteered for one year's service in the Philippines. When he got to Manila, he found a cholera epidemic raging through the city. Dr. Zeller's year of service came and went, but his sense of duty kept him overseas. The epidemic finally burned itself out at the end of August 1902, and Dr. Zeller was released from his army service. He arrived home late in October 1902, and took charge of the asylum on November 1.

The asylum, which had opened in Dr. Zeller's absence on February 10, 1902, was not at all what Zeller had expected. In the first place, not a single one of the 690 patients had come to the asylum from the almshouses of the state – as specifically required by the law authorizing the asylum's founding. Secondly, the asylum was more like a prison than a medical institution, with heavy bars on the windows and doors, and many patients restrained in straitjackets, handcuffs, shackles, and the like, and kept behind locked doors.

Dr. Zeller immediately set out to change all this.

When the Peoria Women's Club needed a superintendent to oversee the newly founded asylum in Bartonville, Dr. Zeller returned to his childhood stomping grounds. His stewardship of the asylum was a natural next step.

Zeller was trained as a physician, not as a psychiatrist. He took the Hippocratic Oath very seriously – "First, do no harm". That's the way he approached patient care – with common sense, not hidebound ways of treating the insane.

The insane were often considered dangerous, prone to fits of madness and violence. Thus it was assumed they had to be restrained. Dr. Zeller writes of this in his autobiography.

> "No one in this comparatively new country ⟦meaning Illinois⟧ was deemed capable of managing an asylum for the insane. They must draw their talent from the Eastern states, and did. Security was their only thought and the result was that for two human generations every abomination that usage had established as necessary in caring for these unfortunates was continued ...Why, only a few years ago when one hundred patients were being transferred to Peoria from another institution, the attendants were told as the train was nearing us 'hurry and remove all restraint, those fellows down there don't tolerate it and will ridicule us'. We got the 100 patients and they ⟦the attendants⟧ returned with two large chests filled with sole leather anklets, wristlets and strait jackets, and that superintendent was deemed one of the ablest in the country. He could thrill a woman's club audience or high school class with brilliant discourses on psychoanalysis but they never get to see the apparently heartless methods he tolerated in his institution."

Dr. Zeller started shaking things up even before he took the job of superintendent. In 1897, he took a tour of the hilltop in preparation for taking the reins. At that point in time, most institutions were built on the Kirkbride plan – one massive building that housed all of the patients. The Kirkbride plan had its advantages – a central location, adequate fresh air for the patients housed there – but Dr. Zeller realized there were better ways of housing the asylum's patients.

And this Kirkbride building in particular was dismally unsuited for housing *any* patients. The ground of the bluff overlooking the Illinois River is honeycombed with ravines and natural springs. In addition, the area where the asylum was being built had previously been mined for the coal abundant at that spot along the river. Rumor had it that the building's contractors were shady characters, with ties to the mob – the mob that would in a few decades make Chicago, three hours north of Bartonville, a hotbed of organized crime.

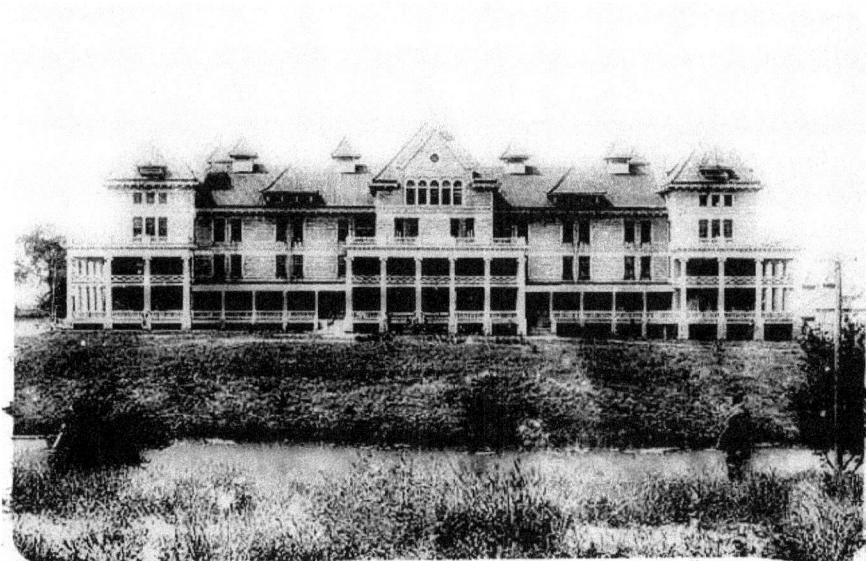

The Illinois Hospital for the Incurable opened in 1902 after its design was approved by Dr. Zeller.

As Dr. Zeller inspected the building – a building that was due to welcome its first patients within weeks – he noted the crumbling foundation, the shoddy materials that made up the walls (which were already beginning to buckle under the weight of the massive building), the utter lack of ventilation and natural light. He refused to sign off on the building. Instead, he insisted it be torn down.

When the Illinois Hospital for the Incurable Insane opened its doors on February 10, 1902, it was built to Dr. Zeller's specifications. Patients were housed in cottages, according to their afflictions. Alcoholics, schizophrenics, epileptics, army veterans suffering from shell shock, all were grouped together, living in their own cottage. Each cottage was overseen by a married couple who served as caretakers, giving the asylum a feel of home. Patients found refuge in being surrounded by others who were suffering the same way. Successful treatment soared. Many patients emerged from the asylum cured, despite the institution's name.

In fact, that was Zeller's entire philosophy. In 1907, he spoke before the Illinois senate, requesting that they change the name of his asylum. "Don't tell my patients they're incurable," he insisted. "I'm here to do just that." In 1907, the name of the institution was changed to the Illinois General Hospital for the Insane, and in 1909, it was changed again, to the Peoria State Hospital.

The mission statement of the asylum was simple. Dr. Zeller and his staff believed in treating patients with kindness. Zeller had the bars removed from the windows of all of the asylum buildings, famously repurposing them into animal cages for a small zoo on the grounds. He had his staff collect the straitjackets and manacles the asylum had originally been equipped with, and he had them put in a small room next to his office. He kept them as museum pieces, something for his staff to point to and say, "Never again. Not here. Not at this institution."

By the autumn of 1904, eight new cottages had been built and were ready to house new patients. The paint had barely dried when Dr. Zeller began to fill those cottages. He contacted the county judge, requesting the immediate transfer of insane almshouse residents. Dr. Zeller used his authority as superintendent of the state's first long-term care facility to do a lot of good. He took trips all over the state, with one goal: to seek out the most pathetic cases, patients who were undernourished, neglected, possibly being abused in the disinterested care of the almshouses and poor farms.

It was on his visit to the Adams County almshouse that he found Rhoda Derry.

CHAPTER NINETEEN
HER HERO

Dr. Zeller strides along the hallway, listening with half an ear to the nervous chatter of the man who walks next to him. Jacob B. Wolfe is fifty-four years old, less than a decade older than Zeller, but he seems to find the younger man intimidating. He hasn't smiled once since they'd entered the building where the patients were housed.

As if anyone could find anything to smile about in this place, Zeller thinks, but he keeps his grimace of distaste to himself. In the few short years he has been superintendent of the asylum at Bartonville, he has spoiled himself and his staff. The Adams County Poor House is actually one of the best-run poorhouses in the state. It is located on rolling hills, with a good water supply and good drainage for that water. Still, there has to be a reason Superintendent Wolfe has only two employees – a matron and an insane servant girl – to care for the physical and emotional needs of some one hundred and fifty inmates. Whether that reason was lack of funds, sheer ignorance, or willful cussedness, remains to be seen.

"And in here – well, I suppose I'll let you see for yourself," Wolfe says, gesturing Zeller before him into the next room. The room is much the same as the others – bare white walls, a closed window looking out onto treetops just beginning to show the colors of fall, a faint reek of piss in the air – but rather than two cots in the room, there is only one. A naked woman slumps on the cot, peering with bleary eyes at the two men. Wolfe nods at the woman, a brief acknowledgement. But Zeller's attention is drawn by the box bed against the other wall. A canvas sheet is thrown over the box, but a shuffling noise of constant movement comes from under the sheet.

Zeller crouches down next to the box bed, curious about the lumpy shape within. He pulls the stiff cover back just as Wolfe mumbles, "I wouldn't ... I mean, we can hardly keep clothes on her. That robe's all she'll tolerate."

Zeller nods absently. He'd assumed the patient was female from the longish dark hair that clings to her face in lank strands, but experience has taught him that first appearances aren't always accurate. He strokes the matted hair away from her face, trying to uncover her eyes, to meet her gaze.

His fingers brush against her face with a horrible dipping sensation. Moments later, he is staring into the woman's blank, scarred eye sockets. Twists of old ropy scar tissue crisscross the empty hollows like fleshy spiderwebs.

Eyes are the windows to the soul, but this woman has no eyes.

Dr. Zeller grabs the rough wooden side of the box bed, fighting the urge to reel back in horror. Years of training kick in instantly. A doctor must never react in shock at what he sees, even if the patient is unaware of him.

Zeller has a quick, analytical mind. He had long ago taught himself to see the whole person, to comprehend the glimpses of sanity in a face that showed only the blankness of lunacy. Once upon a time, he can tell, this woman had been beautiful. Once upon a time, she could have gazed back at him.

The woman in the box bed turns her face up to him, nudging her temple against his fingers. Her lips part, and a tiny noise, like the mewl of a kitten, slips out. Something in his heart breaks a little.

"What's her name?"

"Rhoda ... uh, Rhoda Derry."

At the hesitation in Wolfe's voice, Zeller's compassion sours to outrage. He pushes himself up from the box bed and straightens to face the superintendent.

"How long has she been in this state?"

"Uh ... well, I'm not exactly sure," the other man waffles. "I'd have to check the records –"

"How long?" Zeller thunders.

"I don't know, exactly! Years!"

Zeller forces icy control into his voice. "Let's find out, shall we? Let's just go and check those records."

Back in Wolfe's office, Dr. Zeller sits ramrod-straight in the visitor's chair while Wolfe fusses with files. The air in the office still smells faintly of the roast chicken Wolfe's wife had laid on for lunch. Portraits of previous superintendents gaze dispassionately down on the two men. Zeller imagines the men themselves, looking down their noses at their inmates with the same utter lack of interest.

The present superintendent's face is ashen as he looks up from the papers. "1860."

Zeller rouses himself from his thoughts. "What?"

"1860. September third. That's when Rhoda was admitted."

Zeller's eyes narrow as he does the math. "Years? Try decades! And has that poor woman been trapped in that box bed the entire time?"

Wolfe's tone of voice is miserable as he replies. "No. According to the records, she was so violent for the first couple of decades she was here, she was confined to a Utica crib. She put her eyes out sometime in the first decade. The records from 1870 say she was blind then."

Zeller feels an unpleasant lurch in the pit of his stomach as the chicken breast and roasted potatoes he'd had for lunch tries to make a repeat appearance. He is familiar with the Utica crib. It is a wooden cage, about two feet high. A violent patient would be locked in this cage, hands tied to his sides, straps around his chest and legs – trapped like an animal. "And she spent how many years in the Utica crib?"

"You have to understand!" Wolfe bursts out. "She's quiet now, but she's violent! She swallows everything we give her to eat, pits, seeds, and all! She'd eat the bones if we gave them to her! If we let her out and she was unattended for even a moment, she'd find something sharp on the floor, a pin, a penny, a nail, and into her mouth it would go. Up until two or three years ago, she'd rip off her clothes during her fits – we had to tie them onto her. It's only been in the past couple of years that she's quieted down enough to keep her clothes on. My god, man, she clawed her own eyes out! We – they – they had to keep her locked in a crib."

Dr. Zeller runs a shaking hand down over the brush of his mustache. "Had to ..." He sits up even straighter in his chair.

"She's coming with me."

Jacob Wolfe's color goes from panic-white to the dull-brick flush of angry embarrassment. His lips tighten as his gaze locks in helpless fury on his superior. "You can't do that. What if ... people will blame me. People will think my almshouse let her get ... that way."

Dr. Zeller feels his face settle into what his wife Sophie calls his "military man" expression. "Either Rhoda Derry comes with me, or I shut your institution down, effective immediately. Then who will people blame?"

He leans forward. "If you treated a dog like that, you'd be in jail for cruelty. You do realize that, don't you?"

Wolfe's eyes widen as the threat sinks home. "No other institution would want her. Any inspection finding an inmate in that condition ... can you imagine the blame? She's a wreck, utterly broken. There's no fixing her. No other facility would take that responsibility."

Zeller stands. "Well then, I count myself fortunate that my asylum is like no other facility."

The train from Quincy is delayed the evening of September 26, 1904. There is a washout on the tracks, so the train pulls into the station at the top of the hill in Bartonville very late – around one in the morning. The sixty patients being transferred from the Adams County Poor House are huddled in a boxcar, crowded together for warmth in the chilly night air. Nurses and attendants meet the train, ready to escort the new patients up the gentle slope of the hill to the new C Row cottages.

The attendants from Adams County cast a critical eye over their charges, looking them over once more. Everyone who comes to the Illinois Hospital for the Incurable Insane knows what a stickler old Dr. Zeller is, how he hates to see any patient in chains. That was how he had amassed his collection, by confiscating any shackles that arrived on the patients. Those shackles cost money – the attendants make sure to take them off and hide them well in advance of the train chugging into the station at the top of the hill.

At one end of the boxcar stands an industrial-sized wicker laundry basket. A couple of burly attendants each grab an end of the basket and haul it out of the boxcar. They assume the basket contains the patients' clothing, so they hump it out of the car and set it none too gently on the train station platform. The exhausted group, nurses and patients alike, head up the slope of the hill to the cottages in C Row.

"This seem a bit heavy to you?" one attendant grunts to the other as they lug it.

"Yeah, put it down for a second. I need a break."

The basket hits the ground with a thump, and another sound – an indignant squawk – arises from the pile of clothes. A dingy white gown shifts, pushed aside by a bony hand.

"Gawdamn," one of the attendants breathes. "Nurse! NURSE!"

That night, for the first time in forty-four years, Rhoda Derry sleeps in a bed, with clean white sheets. Strong hands bathe her in warm water, and she smells the pungently antibiotic scent of the soap that washes the filth of years from *her wrinkled skin. Those same hands wrap her in a soft towel, drying her until she almost purrs with the unexpected pleasure.*

Then she is lifted, then falling falling falling – until she lands in softness, like a mother's arms. She turns her head, and her nose bumps smoothness. She sniffs – the memory is faint, but still there, buried deep in her mind. That is the scent of a clean pillowcase, taken from the line only hours before. Rhoda imagines she can still feel the sunshine that had warmed the cotton.

It has been so long since she's cried. Her last tears had been torrents of frustration, salty acid burning the bloody ruined sockets. Now she feels hot tears once again – of relief, of grief for all the wasted years. Wetness slides across unfeeling hollows, then traces hot, wet trails down her temples. She sobs aloud until a gentle female voice starts to croon a lullaby. A soft touch wipes the tears away. "Hushabye, don't you cry ..." The voice cracks, then steadies.

Rhoda Derry sleeps.

CHAPTER TWENTY
RHODA AT THE PEORIA STATE HOSPITAL

During the summer of 1904, builders were hard at work on the grounds of the asylum, completing the cottages of C Row, on the east side of the crest of the hill.

The new buildings provided living quarters for hundreds more patients. Before they opened, patients were temporarily housed in two of the older buildings. The general store provided shelter for a hundred and fifty male patients. And female patients – 128 of them – were housed in the "employee's building", which would much later become known as the Bowen Building. When the C Row cottages were finished, the patients were moved into their new homes.

This 1904 expansion of the asylum at Bartonville was a godsend to other institutions. Even before the asylum opened in 1902, the superintendents of other facilities were making lists of patients they planned to send to Bartonville. It is possible Jacob Wolfe had planned to send Rhoda north all along. The fact that the Illinois Hospital for the Incurable Insane was planned as a long-term care facility right from the jump was a powerful draw. This was something new for Illinois, and it was desperately needed. Not only would this facility provide long-term care for the insane who needed it, it would also ease the pressure on other facilities around the state. If one person takes up a bed in an asylum for, say, fifty years, in that time you can help hundreds of patients who might only need to stay for several months at a time. Most institutions were not designed for long-term care.

Dr. Zeller was not unaware of Rhoda. He received copies of the state's annual reports on the almshouses. He was in contact with the superintendents of these almshouses, including Jacob Wolfe. Zeller was perfectly aware that his new institution was going to be home to the worst of the worst cases from all over the state. He had designed it that way. He wanted those patients. But he had the sneaking suspicion that the trainloads of patients that were showing up almost daily were simply patients the other institutions didn't want. This frustrated him: Zeller firmly believed that no patient was incurable. But how could he prove this point if he wasn't allowed to care for the most wretched, pathetic cases?

Being a military man, Dr. Zeller resolved to take matters into his own hands. Rather than allowing the superintendents of the other institutions to make the decisions for him, he went to the almshouses himself. He wanted to ensure that his hospital was, in fact, taking on the worst of the worst.

Jacob Wolfe wrote to Dr. Zeller when the asylum in Bartonville opened. Zeller's reply was swift and emphatic: "Send her along, God bless her." Certainly, Zeller would have known of Rhoda's situation, or his reply wouldn't have been so decisive. But we do also know that Dr. Zeller did visit the Adams County almshouse, and found Rhoda there. For some reason, the transfer didn't take place. The discussion between Zeller and Wolfe was never documented, but employees of the almshouse gossiped. Apparently there was some sort of argument between the two superintendents over Rhoda's situation. Perhaps Dr. Zeller's "send her along, God bless her" was a pleasant fiction made up for the newspapers, to hide Zeller's fury at Rhoda's condition.

Dr. Zeller was highly conscious of the power of the press, and he used it to his institution's advantage. It is entirely possible that he tipped off the papers in September 1904, when Rhoda was released from the almshouse. The Quincy Daily Whig reported Rhoda's move to Bartonville with the blaring headline "Renews Stories of Witchcraft", and the Quincy Daily Journal took up the tale as well. The papers got their information from Benjamin Bragg, a Lima resident who had known the Derrys since 1851 – he actually lived in their former home. The attorney who drew up the papers for Rhoda's removal from the almshouse, James N. Sprigg, had asked Bragg for information about Rhoda's life, and the papers picked up on this knowledgeable source. Bragg recounted the story of Rachel shooting at imaginary witches in the Derry house. The newspapers ate up the ghoulish story with relish, but Dr. Zeller accomplished his goal; he drew people's attention to the plight of the mentally ill, and in doing so, he got publicity for the asylum.

In preparation for opening the asylum, the institution arranged to use the railroad spur that ended at the top of the hill. The spur divided into two tracks just before the crest of the hill. When Dr. Zeller laid out the plans for the asylum grounds, he put the train station next to the north side track, and the general store next to the south side track, for ease of delivery. Trains carrying patients were routed onto the north track, and supplies for the asylum, to the south track. The power house was also on the north side of the track, and that's where deliveries of coal were dropped off.

This railroad spur made it easy for the asylum to welcome patients who came from other institutions. Almshouses, and other asylums, simply loaded their patients onto a train and sent them to Bartonville. The patients were met at the station and escorted to whatever cottage they were assigned to.

We know from his writings, and from the admiration of his contemporaries, that Dr. George Zeller was a compassionate, caring superintendent of the Peoria State Hospital. It's said he was "a military man to his employees, and a father figure to his patients". Indeed, he and Sophie never did have children. They considered the patients of the asylum their children.

Dr. Zeller took that responsibility – the continued care of his children – very seriously. He was adamant about training his staff to his own specifications. He refused to hire any nurses or attendants who had previously been employed at another institution. (He derisively called them "bug-housers".) He figured – and he was undoubtedly right – that other asylums wouldn't hold their staff to as high a code of conduct as he planned to do. He preferred to train his own staff from the ground up, to his own exacting standards. If somehow a staff member did slip past, having worked at another asylum in the past, and Dr. Zeller found out about the oversight, he would fire that employee immediately and without cause.

His staff shared his dedication. Surely, the nurses at the asylum knew what they had signed on for when they applied to work with Dr. Zeller. They knew the asylum would be taking in the worst of the worst, cases from the dregs of the state's almshouses. It was right there, in the institution's first name – The Illinois Hospital for the Incurable Insane. But even that knowledge couldn't have prepared them for Rhoda's arrival.

Jacob Wolfe, the superintendent of the Adams County Poor Farm, would have had an excellent point – had Rhoda been found at *any* institution, having survived for over four decades in her wretched condition, the staff of that facility certainly would have been blamed for the squalor she'd endured for so long.

And that, precisely, is why Dr. Zeller spent so much time in his capacity as superintendent of the Peoria State Hospital visiting almshouses and poor farms. He made a career out of searching out the inmates who were suffering the most. He took these wretched people to the asylum and cared for them – not only because he cared for them as patients, but also because he genuinely believed the Peoria State Hospital was the finest facility in the world. He used these worst-case scenarios to demonstrate to the nay-sayers what a vitally important service the asylum provided. Rhoda Derry was simply one of the first patients to benefit from Zeller's crusade.

When Rhoda arrived at the Peoria State Hospital, she was in surprisingly good shape for having been locked in a cage for forty-four years. Her hair was still dark in spite of her age – she turned seventy several weeks after her arrival at the asylum. The nurses washed it and brushed it, bringing it back to something like luster.

But her body showed signs of her incredible ordeal. She had gone in to the almshouse a young woman of twenty-six. Now she was seventy years old. Her collarbone had been broken in several places. Her eyes were long gone. She had beaten her teeth in years before. And she couldn't tell anyone at the asylum how it had happened, or what led her to this grievous self-harm. She'd done it to herself. That was all.

Rhoda had little medical care in the almshouse. It's a miracle she survived, but she did. She survived the horrific damage she did to herself by clawing her eyes out. An infection from filthy fingernails could easily have traveled to her brain and killed her. She also survived whatever infection may have stolen her power of speech. Mentally, emotionally, she was broken beyond repair. But physically, she was still a strong, healthy woman, at least for the first few years she was at the almshouse. She couldn't do anything about the deterioration of her hips that eventually robbed her of her mobility. But her body survived.

In his letter to the judge of the Adams County Court, written to inform the court of Rhoda's death, Dr. Zeller wrote, "We never allowed her to become the object of curiosity, but when real students of social problems came along, we took them to the bedside of Rhody and her case alone called down more blessings upon the State than all the eighteen hundred others we are now caring for. No one ever blamed the alms house authorities for her former care and all seemed to feel that they gave her the best they could afford and I often told them that fact that she had been kept alive all those years proved that she was not without considerate care, but somehow visitors went away with the feeling that this one case alone justified the erection of this institution and no person ever saw her without becoming a firm convert to the belief in state care of the insane."

If there is just a whiff of "doth protest too much" in these words, I think we can forgive Dr. Zeller his zeal. Insane asylums have always had an appalling reputation. Stories of abuse are shared with ghoulish relish. We've seen the wretched conditions of some of the almshouses. People who had family members with mental illness often cared for them at home for as long as they could. Unfortunately, without proper treatment, the mania or depression became so entrenched in the victim's mind that they became deeply afflicted, sometimes to the point of endangering the family members who were trying to protect them.

Dr. Zeller and the staff of the Peoria State Hospital worked tirelessly to change this attitude towards mental illness. The asylum was the most modern state-funded institution in the country for many, many years. Dr. Zeller gave free run of the hospital grounds to any politician, member of the press, or ordinary citizen who cared to visit. This open-door policy was meant to reassure the public that everything possible was being done to care for the insane in a modern, compassionate way.

Rhoda became famous – not only locally but *world-famous* – as "the patient who was brought here in a basket". But Dr. Zeller never allowed her to be gawked at by curiosity seekers. The staff who cared for Rhoda Derry did so at Dr. Zeller's insistence, so that no one could blame the Peoria State Hospital for her condition.

And care for her they did. As the asylum grew in resources, and in popularity, Rhoda benefitted from the three farms that supplied the patients with three meals a day of locally-grown food. Knowing Rhoda's excruciating history, the nurses doted on her. They kept her happy and entertained. They fed her nutritious food with tender care. They changed her bedsheets the moment she soiled them. Even the smallest kindnesses were acts of unspeakable generosity for Rhoda, who had known only neglect for decades.

Rhoda became a daughter of the institution. She could no longer see, but the nurses made sure she experienced the hilltop in any way that was still available to her. They dragged a mattress out to the porch of the cottage in which she lived, and let her sit out in the fresh air. They let her sit in the gardens that dotted the grounds, and feel the sun on her face, and hear the birds chirping, and smell the flowers whose colors she couldn't see. They brought her to dances – ragtime would have made its way to Peoria by that time, so maybe Rhoda swayed her wasted body and clapped her gnarled hands to the snappy beat of the Maple Leaf Rag or The Entertainer.

Rhoda lived in her C Row cottage for less than two years. In the first half of 1906, she developed full-blown tuberculosis. She most likely picked up the disease in the almshouse – and she was incredibly lucky that it took its time progressing. Medical care was available to almshouse inmates, but it was cursory at best.

The staff of the Peoria State Hospital, on the other hand, had plenty of experience in caring for tuberculosis patients. TB was a problem on the hilltop almost from the opening day. The original buildings of the asylum included two hospitals, one for routine medical care, and one for surgery. But the tuberculosis cases soon overran the Michell Hospital's capacity. Patients suffering from "the white plague" were housed in tent colonies, exposed to plenty of fresh air. But even the beds in the tents weren't enough. The tents, originally designed for temporary open-air therapy during good weather, had to be pressed into service year-round. Stoves were moved into the tents, and the asylum made the patients as comfortable as possible. Overcrowding in these tent colonies led to the asylum receiving grants to build two tuberculosis hospitals in 1922.

But 1922 was still far off. In 1906, patients suffering from acute TB were housed, for lack of any other space at the time, in Dining Hall A. When Rhoda began to show signs of TB, she was moved from her cottage to a bed in Dining Hall A. She was probably there for a matter of months as her disease progressed.

And it was there that she took her final gasping breath. She died on October 9, 1906, the day before she would have turned seventy-two.

The nurses responsible for her care were devastated. Far from being relieved that their burden was gone, they shed tears for the broken old woman who had left them too soon.

Here, at last, we come to the final mystery of Rhoda's life. There are four cemeteries on the hilltop. Two of the cemeteries were started at the same time, at the very beginning of the asylum's history. Cemetery One was for folks whose families had money to bury them in relative style. There are more headstones here with names on them, memorials to family members who passed on, no matter that they died in an institution.

Cemetery Two, on the other hand, was the paupers' burying ground. The patients who died at the asylum whose bodies went unclaimed for burial in family plots were laid to rest here, in graves unmarked except for the identification number that had been issued to them when they entered the asylum. There are a few headstones here, but they are obviously later additions, placed there (and paid for) by family members a generation or two later, descendants who aren't as embarrassed to admit that a relative of theirs died in an asylum.

So why was Rhoda buried in Cemetery One? At the time of her death, she had outlived nearly all of her relatives. Only her brother, James McCann

Derry, was still alive from her generation. She did have a nephew, Levi Slater, who lived in the Quincy area. But as far as we know, none of her relatives ever came to visit her, either in the almshouse or at the Peoria State Hospital. So who was responsible for having her buried in the more respectable cemetery, rather than the potter's field?

I think the answer lies, yet again, with Dr. Zeller and his staff. Rhoda was not only an object lesson in how to treat the insane. She was also a cherished patient. When she died, she got a family's respect ... something she had been denied for most of her life.

Rhoda had a special relationship with Dr. Zeller. Even without sight, with a mind ravaged by grief and decades of imprisonment, still she knew absolutely who had saved her. Perhaps she recognized his voice, or maybe she smelled his cologne. But whenever Dr. Zeller walked into the room, Rhoda lit up. It's said she never smiled – except when George Zeller came into the room.

At some point, someone – probably Dr. Zeller, with his eye for promotion – decided to take Rhoda's picture. We should be very grateful for this, as it is the only known photograph of Rhoda Derry. In it, she is crouched on the floor, her skinny legs drawn up in front of her, all knobby kneecaps and bone. Her claw-like hands clutch and scrabble at nothing on the floor in front of her. Her hair, still mostly dark at seventy-one (as far as we can tell from a black-and-white photograph), is cut in a short hairdo that actually looks somewhat styled. It was standard procedure to crop the long hair of female tuberculosis patients, as the TB germs are carried on the hair and clothing. The length of her hair seems to suggest that Rhoda's hair had been cut short just a few weeks before the photo was taken. So it may have been made sometime in the late summer of 1906, when Rhoda was moved from her cottage to Dining Hall A.

But look again – look close. The crude camera of 1906 can't snap a crisp, focused picture, because Rhoda is always in motion. But her toothless mouth is open, and the lips curl upward in what looks like a grin. She is *beaming*. Her expression, as far as we can tell through the blur, is bright and engaged.

Rhoda actually looks happy.

Is Dr. Zeller in the room somewhere, maybe behind the photographer, a little off to his right? That's where Rhoda is facing, like a flower following the sun. Rhoda had severely limited mobility, but when Dr. Zeller was around, she roused herself enough to crab on her gnarled hands across the floor and reach up to tug on his pants leg.

After decades of misery, Rhoda finally found her hero.

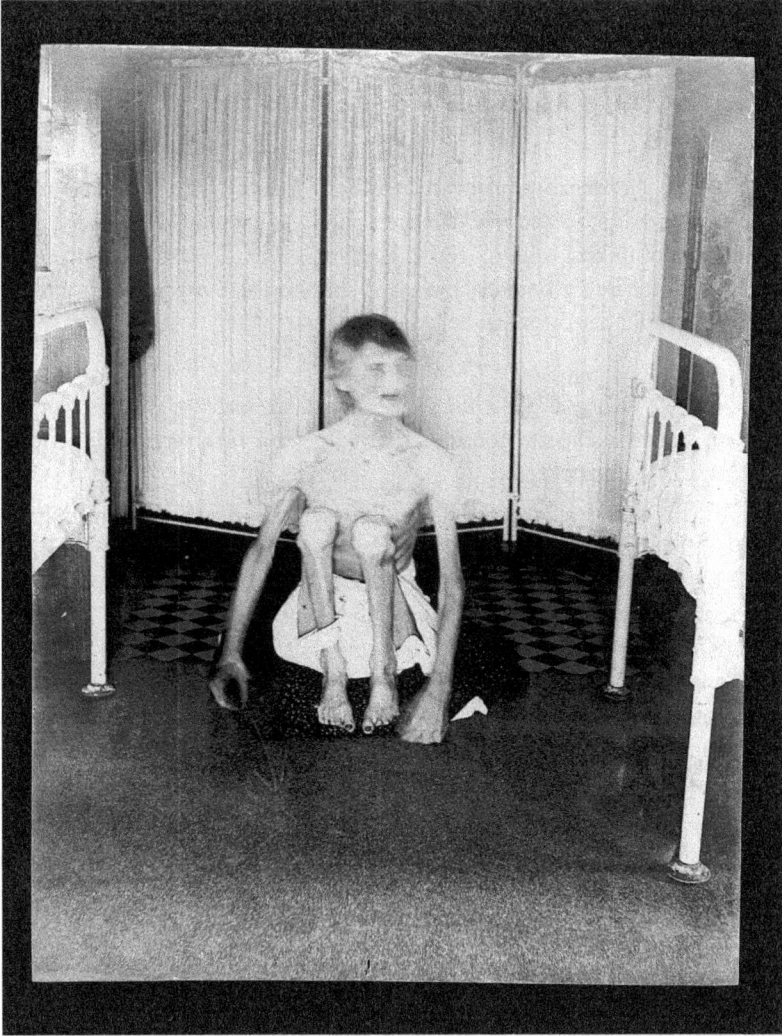

CHAPTER TWENTY-ONE
THE DIAGNOSIS

Here's the question many people have asked over the years: what was going on in Rhoda's spectacularly damaged mind? What was wrong with her that the top asylum of its day couldn't fix? If Jacob and Rachel were to stuff themselves and their daughter into a time machine, and show up at a psych ward with Rhoda in tow, what would her diagnosis be?

In 1656, Georg Tross, a minister in England, wrote about his own mental breakdown. Modern experts consider this to be the first written description of what we now call schizophrenia.

When considering possibilities for Rhoda's diagnosis, schizophrenia is usually the first answer that gets tossed into the ring. In the late nineteenth century, this was known as dementia praecox. The "praecox" part comes from Latin, and basically means "early" – it's the same root that gives us the word "precocious". If a patient appeared to have dementia – a disorder of the elderly – but wasn't in fact old, they were diagnosed with dementia praecox. (Rhoda would probably not ever have picked up this label. Dementia praecox was first described by Emil Kraeplin around 1893, far too late to have been applied to Rhoda. By 1893, everyone had long since given up pinning a diagnosis on her.)

Symptoms of schizophrenia include audio and visual hallucinations and delusional thinking. It's a chronic mental disorder that affects how the patient thinks, feels, and behaves toward others. A patient with schizophrenia has trouble distinguishing between reality and what's going on in his own mind.

Signs of schizophrenia may appear abruptly, or they may develop over months or even years. Some signs include hearing or seeing things that aren't there, a feeling of being watched, speaking or writing nonsense, a change in personality, withdrawal from social situations, irrational, angry or fearful response to loved ones, an inability to sleep or concentrate, and extreme preoccupation with religion or the occult.

The patient may suffer delusions that people are spying on them, or that they are someone famous. Auditory hallucinations, in particular hearing voices giving commands, are common. The schizophrenic might display disordered thinking, which erupts in nonsensical speech, jumping from one topic to another, even making up their own random sounds.

At first blush, schizophrenia seems like a fairly logical diagnosis for Rhoda. Her insistence that "Old Scratch" was after her certainly seems to fit with an extreme preoccupation with the occult. And her hallucinations of witches flying around the house are held up as evidence of a schizophrenia diagnosis.

But it doesn't really fit. For one thing, the average age of onset for schizophrenia is late teens or early twenties for men, and late twenties or early thirties for women, although it can begin at even older ages. Rhoda had her first break with reality in her late teens – that's awfully early for the onset of schizophrenia in a woman. Also, the voices that schizophrenics usually hear tend to be commanding or belittling. We have no evidence that Rhoda heard voices that told her to do things, or voices that told her she was worthless.

Another possible diagnosis is epilepsy, specifically temporal lobe epilepsy. Given Rhoda's condition after decades in the almshouse – a collarbone that had been broken more than once, teeth beaten in by her own hands – some sort of seizure disorder seems logical. Also, if we look at the records saying that Rhoda "beat her own eyes out", and interpret that as the result of flailing fists rather than clawing fingers, seizures seem even more likely.

Temporal lobe epilepsy causes, among other things, feelings of unexplainable panic, and preoccupation with philosophical concerns. Might this be an explanation for Rhoda's first breakdown, when she said "Old Scratch" was after her?

But again, there was so much more going on in Rhoda's shattered mind. The violent rages, the hallucinations, the psychic prescience, all of the *weirdness* just can't be explained by TLE, or any other form of epilepsy.

So what the hell *was* wrong with Rhoda Derry?

At the time, Rhoda's affliction was blamed pretty squarely on witchcraft. (This wasn't her only diagnosis. Dr. H. O. Collins, the physician for the Adams County almshouse, mentioned in his report for the September 1904 term that Rhoda's troubles were supposedly caused by "suppression of the menses", an all-too-common catchall phrase slapped on women who were being obstreperous.) Yes, Illinois' first mental hospital, at Jacksonville, had opened its doors not ten years before, in 1851. At the time, it was the most modern mental health care facility in the state, and one of the best in the nation. The doctors there would have sniffed at such a backward theory of mental illness. But even the staff at Jacksonville encountered ... oddities ... when caring for Rhoda. When she was released as incurable, and went home to two more years of inexplicable events, her family was at a loss. Witchcraft could start to seem like a reasonable diagnosis, or at least an explanation.

After all, for centuries before Rhoda's birth, most insanity had been blamed on witchcraft or demonic possession. Rhoda's own grandmother, Moll Derry, might even have leaned toward the demonic possession theory. Rhoda's life was so littered with the strange and the outright bizarre – even flavored with a dollop of the supernatural for a little extra spice – that it is immensely difficult to pin down her situation with a modern diagnosis. But it's worth a try.

I believe Rhoda Derry suffered from adjustment disorder. A person with adjustment disorder develops emotional and behavioral symptoms as a reaction to a stressful event. Because people with this condition often have some of the same symptoms of clinical depression such as crying jags, loss of interest in daily activities, or feelings of hopelessness, adjustment disorder is sometimes informally called "situational depression". Unlike major depression, though, adjustment disorder doesn't involve as severe a response to stress, such as suicidal thinking or behavior.

The specific diagnostic criteria for adjustment disorder, according to the American Psychiatric Association's Diagnostic and Statistical Manual, Fifth Edition (familiarly known as the DSM-V), are these:

> Emotional or behavioral symptoms develop in response to an identifiable stressor within three months of the onset of the stressor plus either one or both of 1) marked distress that is out of proportion to the severity or intensity of the stressor, and/or 2) significant impairment in social, occupational or other areas of functioning;
>
> the stress-related disturbance does not meet criteria for another mental disorder and is not merely an exacerbation of a preexisting mental disorder; and, the symptoms do not represent normal bereavement.

This fits Rhoda's situation to a tee. Nancy's threat of a curse was the stressor. Rhoda's overreaction could be considered out of proportion to the severity of the stressor.

The disorder is a pathological extreme of what is otherwise a normal coping process. Adjustment disorder is primarily treated with psychotherapy, although in some cases medication may also be prescribed to alleviate symptoms. It's been found that talk therapy is extremely effective in treating adjustment disorder. A therapist might encourage the patient to express emotions in a safe environment, or gently point out that the patient's reaction is blown all out of proportion to the situation. The therapist may suggest healthier ways of dealing with stressful situations in the future. This approach usually takes care of the issue within a few sessions of treatment.

I spoke with Suzanne Stambaugh, Psy.D., who works at PsychARTS in Austin, Texas. She walked me through the DSM-V description of adjustment disorder, and agreed that this was a possible explanation for Rhoda's condition.

"It's thought of as a temporary thing. Sometimes, though, it can become permanent." Adjustment disorder that persists in spite of talk therapy may progress into a more serious mental condition. The DSM-V agrees: studies suggest that adults with adjustment disorder have a good long-term prognosis, while adolescents may eventually develop major psychiatric conditions.

Nowadays, in addition to treating adjustment disorder with talk therapy, doctors can use a pharmacological component. Pharmacotherapy involves benzodiazepenes or plant extracts, such as kava kava or valerian. All of these serve as relaxants, and are used mostly to improve coping skills by moderating symptoms like insomnia or anxiety. With those stressors out of the way, the patient can focus on getting better. Psychotherapy is considered to be much more effective, though.

Interestingly, talk therapy was the main course of treatment at the Illinois State Hospital for the Insane. Even in the middle of the nineteenth century, doctors realized the value of talking through one's issues.

But here is part of Rhoda's tragedy: if adjustment disorder lasts longer than six months or so, it can become permanent. Rhoda's break with reality happened around 1852, and she wasn't admitted to Jacksonville until 1856. She spent four years in misery, aching with her need for Charles, cowering in terror as Rachel fired a pistol in the house at invisible witches. She refused to see Nancy Phenix, even when Nancy tried to explain that the "curse" was nothing more than a ruse. Heaven knows where Charles was at this point. If Rhoda had been taken to Jacksonville right away, within six months of her confrontation with Nancy, maybe the talk therapy at the hospital could have helped her. At this distance, it's impossible to say for sure.

There's another component to consider when looking at a possible diagnosis: Rhoda's seizures. The interesting thing about adjustment disorder is that having it does not preclude the patient developing other disorders.

Psychogenic non-epileptic seizures usually develop in young women in their late teens and early twenties. They are often brought on by psychological stress. Patients who experience PNES often also suffer from depression and anxiety, which contribute to the emotional stress.

According to the Epilepsy Foundation, PNES are attacks that may look like epileptic seizures, but are not caused by abnormal brain electrical discharges. Patients suffering from PNES may look like they are experiencing convulsions similar to tonic clonic seizures, with shaking and falling (as opposed to absence seizures, where a patient shows a temporary loss of attention, simply staring off into the distance).

Here's where it gets really interesting. Many patients with PNES have experienced a specific traumatic event, great loss, or sudden change, which led to the appearance of the seizures. PNES – *psychogenic* non-epileptic seizures – are a physical manifestation of a psychological disturbance. They're a type of conversion disorder – meaning that the physical symptoms, the seizures, arise from psychological conflict. The emotional stress is converted into symptoms that look like a neurological disorder. But the seizures actually don't have an organic cause. Conversion disorders tend to develop during adolescence or early adulthood, and they appear to be somewhat more common among women.

So when Derry family lore speaks of Rhoda "spinning around on her head like a top", it is possible that this unusual turn of phrase describes the erratic twists and contortions of a young woman in the throes of a seizure. And the broken collarbone and knocked-out teeth that Dr. Zeller noted upon Rhoda's arrival at the Peoria State Hospital could have been caused by Rhoda's own flailing fists during a convulsion.

We have to remember that especially at a distance of a hundred and fifty years or so, it is nearly impossible to pin down one or two things that neatly explain why Rhoda suffered the way she did. Any diagnosis is just a way to describe how the brain's chemistry has gone awry. Most mental illness is the interplay between real life and imagination – a disconnect between what the mind perceives as reality, and what's actually happening. The chasm between perception and life experience is what we need to focus on, no matter what we end up calling it. Whatever label we use, we can't forget that it was Rhoda's experience that formed her.

Whatever a patient's diagnosis in the middle of the nineteenth century, whether it was dementia, or insanity, or failure in business, or suppression of the menses, it was all treated with talk therapy. There's something to be said for just sitting down with someone who is willing to listen with a sympathetic ear as you pour out all your troubles – even if they're being paid to do it.

And for a long time, that was all there was. About a hundred and ten years separated the opening of the first state hospital in 1851 and the discovery of psychotropic drugs in the 1960s. For more than a century, that was the only real option for humane treatment of the insane: let them talk it out. Maybe they'll get better. Maybe they won't.

The staff at the Illinois State Hospital for the Insane did their best. But their best just wasn't good enough, and it was rendered far too late for Rhoda Derry. If Rhoda had had the opportunity to talk to caring professionals right away, within months or weeks of her break, could she have pulled out of her tailspin? Could she have recovered from the loss of her first love? Could she have gone on to live a normal life, met someone new, gotten married, had children?

We will never know.

INTERLUDE
JANUARY 3, 1974

Dorothy sits at the dining room table, writing in her journal, idly tracing the decorative groove in the wood that runs the length of the table. Her fingers find the nicks and scratches that tell of the furniture's long years of service. It's late, nearly one in the morning, yet she isn't at all sleepy. Bone-tired, sure, but not sleepy. She sighs, and takes another drink of diet soda.

She studies the pills that sit next to the glass, lined up like tiny bullets. Vistaril, to make her relax. Librium, to calm the screaming in her mind. And the ever-present Noludar, which makes her feel so sleepy – but which does nothing for the nightmares that come when she does sleep.

Her hand hovers over the four Noludar tablets. Should she really take them now, with David out of the house and the two little girls asleep upstairs? If she doesn't take them now, she'll be up until dawn. Then the kids will be awake all day, and she'll be useless at caring for them, even with David's help. And David has to get his sleep sometime too. If he didn't have to work that third-shift job and spend so much time in classes, they could all sleep at night ...

She sweeps all nine of the pills into her hand and tosses them back. Grimacing at the bitter taste, she washes them down with a gulp of diet soda.

Dorothy sits for a moment, eyes closed, waiting for the familiar drug-dump feeling. She's done this nearly every night for the past several years. It's just a matter of getting the right dosage and combination of meds – finding which pills will let her sleep without nightmares, which pills will let her be awake during the day to care for her children, which pills will quiet the screaming in her mind. She'll get there someday. By the grace of her God, she'll get there.

The Noludar has started to kick in. If she wants to get the garbage taken out tonight, she'd better do it now. She stands, gripping the solidly comforting wooden edge of the table for a moment. The wooziness passes, and she heads into the kitchen.

The paper bag from Dominick's grocery is nearly full. Dorothy pulls it out, shakes a fresh bag open, pushes it into the can. Then she grabs the full bag and heads for the back door. It's the beginning of January, but she won't need a coat. She's just going to run out to the garbage can, dump the full bag in, and return to the warmth of the house.

When Billie Jean King beat Bobby Riggs in tennis on September 20, 1973, Virginia Slims cigarette ads crowed in jubilation, "You've come a long way, baby!" But women still had a long way to go.

In their January 1960 issue, *Mademoiselle* encouraged its readers to do anything they wanted ... within the parameters of what had already been established as "women's work". In those days, most girls grew to adulthood without ever seeing a woman doctor, lawyer, college professor, police officer, or bus driver. Once *Mademoiselle* finished urging its readers to shoot for the stars, it came back down to earth pretty quickly. A few issues later, the magazine celebrated the end of the school year with an article on careers that focused mostly on secretarial duties. The editors wrapped up the article with a roundup of "pre-job hand-beautifying" tips for the new crop of typists. Women were regularly paid a lower wage than men, and newspapers even had separate classified sections: Help Wanted – Men and Help Wanted – Women.

The middle of the nineteenth century, when Rhoda was struggling with her demons, was a time of great strides forward for young women, but a time of great upheaval too. Young women of the antebellum period had increasing opportunities to work outside the home, and they took those jobs – even if they were simply factory drudgery, maid's work, or teaching. Along with this newfound freedom came, paradoxically, greater strictures on that freedom.

My mother, Dorothy Jeanne McClaren Zethmayr, came of age in the mid-twentieth century, a hundred years after Rhoda. She, along with many other young women of her generation, faced an entirely new set of paradoxes.

In 1950, while in her eighties, Margaret Sanger raised $150,000 for research to create the first human birth control pill. In 1960, Enovid was approved by the FDA for use in the United States. For the first time, women had a convenient, nonintrusive method of birth control available to them, one for which they did not have to depend on men. Soon after that, the number of partners available to use this freedom with dropped precipitously. Young men were being drafted and sent to Vietnam.

The Summer of Love heated things up in 1967. Shaggy guys in bell bottoms and long-haired girls in peasant blouses grooved to the music of the Beatles, the Stones, the Grateful Dead, and the Mamas and the Papas.

But all was not ponchos and patchouli. There were 167 urban riots in 1967 alone. The next year, 1968, was the year both Martin Luther King Jr. and Robert Kennedy were assassinated. In the 1960s, there were six major racial explosions just in the city of Chicago, where my parents lived. The news of the rioting must have been terrifying. The mood of the whole nation was nervous, twitchy. For someone like Dorothy, who was having difficulty dealing with the stresses of daily life at the best of times, those days of the late 1960s must have been extremely stressful.

To add to my mother's stress, my father volunteered his medical services at the Black Panthers' free clinic. In 1968, the Illinois chapter of the Black Panthers was formed on the west side of Chicago. It was headed by a charismatic young black man named Fred Hampton. Before he was killed in 1969, Hampton established free breakfast programs for school children, organized the free medical clinic, and brokered a non-aggression pact between some of Chicago's most notorious street gangs. By 1970, People's Free Medical Clinics had become a requirement for every Black Panthers chapter. The free clinic in Chicago was very sophisticated compared to other Black Panther clinics. It boasted a system of triage, several different exam rooms, and the volunteer services of nursing and medical students, my father among them. My dad was happy to contribute to an organization that was doing so much good in the city. But it can't have been easy on my mother.

Gail Collins, author of *When Everything Changed: The Amazing Journey of Women from 1960 to the Present*, writes: "After (World War II), Americans had a powerful and understandable desire to settle down and return to normal. Since they were doing so in an era of incredible economic growth, it was easy to decide that stay-at-home housewives were part of the package." Why work if you don't have to? If a couple can live comfortably on one income instead of two, why not let the woman stay home and keep house?

Even college was mostly seen as yet another avenue toward finding a husband. Young women went to school to earn the proverbial "Mrs." degree. *Newsweek* reported in 1960 that sixty percent of the women who entered college dropped out before graduating, and most of those quit school to get married. This was another result of the post-war economic boom. Families could now afford to send their daughters to college, even if the girls had no intention of using the resulting education.

Then, with the founding of the National Organization for Women (NOW) in 1966, women were encouraged to work outside the home, no matter what their marital status was. The exploding economy meant jobs – lots of them. And women stepped into them. That same year, President Lyndon B. Johnson suggested that businesses consider hiring women to fill their openings. *Time* ran a headline in November 1966 that announced: "A Good Man is Hard to Find – So They Hire Women". Temp agencies boomed, and even companies like Texas Instruments and IBM began actively recruiting female employees.

The late 1960s were a goldmine for women who wanted to work outside the home. But even in the midst of this hiring frenzy, the male-dominated workforce still gave females the hairy eyeball. Modern TV shows like *Mad Men* and *Life on Mars* take perverse, nostalgic pleasure in looking back at this boorish behavior. *Mad Men's* Don Draper makes us cringe today, at least once an episode. And in *Life on Mars*, Detective Sam Tyler, who has inexplicably found himself thrown back in time from 2008 to 1973, is drawn to Annie Norris, the lone female police officer in Tyler's New York City precinct. Annie, played in the American version by Gretchen Mol, is young, pretty, blonde, and just trying to make her way in the boys' club world of New York City cops. Detective Tyler brings a modern perspective to the macho world of the 1970s.

In the 1960s, even the supposedly enlightened world of science fiction reflected this discomfort with women in the workplace. The future, imagined, wasn't terribly different than the present. Even the famously progressive *Star Trek* boldly went where pretty much every man had gone before. One *Trek* episode ("Turnabout Intruder", air date June 3, 1969) featured a woman who was so desperate to become a starship captain that she arranged to have her brain transplanted into Captain Kirk's body. Janice Lester is even referred to as "mentally unstable", when all she wanted was to be the captain of a starship. Her cover was blown when the crew noticed "Kirk" manicuring his nails at the helm of the Enterprise, and breaking down in nervous hysterics at the slightest sign of trouble. (Fans do consider this to be one of the two worst episodes of the classic series, the other being "Spock's Brain".)

My mother held very few jobs, and those only for a matter of weeks. She waitressed for a few days at a restaurant near the Great Lakes Navy Recruit Training Command, where my dad spent some time. Her biggest tip was from him – fifty cents. (In 1962 that was more than it is today.) Later, she held a job long enough to spend a big chunk of the two or three weeks' earnings on a large refrigerator for their second-floor apartment near 71st and Ashland in Chicago. My dad got stuck moving that fridge just a few weeks later, when Dorothy needed another move, this time to the small apartment above the garage at my grandparents' house in the Chicago suburbs. Dorothy was secretary to a group of salesmen in a small, lively company on the southwest side of Chicago or possibly Cicero, along Archer Avenue. Her boss let her go one day without a clear explanation. My dad got the impression that the problem was with Dorothy's lack of social skills. It must have been a quick turnaround in a short time, because when Dad had met the boss earlier, he had seemed highly satisfied with her work.

Then again, she wouldn't have been expected to hold down a full-time job. But my mother remained aloof from the work force not because of society's pressures, and not because she married my father when she was twenty.

My mother didn't work because she was emotionally incapable of holding down a job.

My mother's generation wanted desperately to change the world. People tuned in, turned on, and dropped out. They joined communes and sat in meditation, going within themselves to try to find a solution to the world's suffering, and their own. Their intent was to save the world by saving themselves. Dorothy was no flower child – what she found in her own mind was neither covered in daisies nor patchouli-scented. It was dark and vicious and horrifying.

Carrying the bag of garbage, Dorothy turns the knob of the back door. The metal is cold under her fingers, and she briefly reconsiders going back for her thick sheepskin coat. But it's just a quick trip out to the garbage cans. She'll be back inside and headed upstairs in less than a minute. She'll look in on the sleeping girls, then she'll tuck herself in to wait for her husband. If she's lucky, she'll be asleep before he gets home.

If she's lucky, there won't be any nightmares.

The January night air hits her with the slap of a freezing wet rag across the face. It had snowed a few days before, and the back steps are still slick with ice. Still carrying the Dominick's bag, Dorothy starts down the steps.

Halfway down, she hits an icy patch. Her feet go out from under her. The bag goes flying as she struggles for balance. She lands badly, hitting her head on the top step. She lies, stunned, blinking with the sudden pain.

She's cold, and the wet slush is melting under her thighs. The Noludar is working, though, fuzzing the edges, blunting the cold.

Dorothy closes her eyes.

When I decided to write about my mother's life, I sent out two letters, to people I figured would have known her well. One was to Dorothy's sister Marlys, my Aunt Janie, in California. The other was to my godmother, Slavka Zabrodsky, who now lives in Michigan.

I never heard back from my aunt. To my knowledge, I have only seen her once, when she brought her two younger sons to Illinois for a visit when all of us kids were in early grade school. They were strangers to me then, and they are strangers to me now.

My godmother, on the other hand, called as soon as she got my letter. We spent hours on the phone playing catch-up. She is still vibrant and active at eighty years old. She told me about the plans for her upcoming birthday party, held on Mother's Day. "I'll send you pictures of the party," she promised. "I'm the redhead."

I told her I had some questions about my mother. Luckily for me, Slavka kept a diary. We spent an hour on the phone one evening, me listening as she flipped through the pages, reminiscing as the dates went past.

"Oh yeah, I remember pulling you and Andre [her son] in that little red wagon. You and your sister spent a lot of time at our house." She turned a page.

"Your mom seemed very lonely a lot of the time. Your dad was working, or taking classes, or something, and he'd stay in a rented room near the college. She was alone a lot.

"Monday, September 7, 1970. Surprised by a call from David Zethmayr." My dad, once again, had dropped me off at Slavka's house. I was to be her responsibility for several hours, rather than my mother's.

"September 12. Zs floated in around suppertime." Often, my parents wouldn't tell Slavka where they were going when they dropped me off. They'd just bring me over and leave me with no warning. Slavka said I behaved very well for her, which made me feel good. No one wants to hear they were a bratty kid.

"Dorothy was such a sweet-natured person." Slavka said my mother was a gentle soul with a great sense of humor. "She smiled a lot."

When my parents met Slavka, she was working part-time as a psychiatric counselor. "I think she was overmedicated when I first met her. There was something about her eyes that was just ..." Her voice trailed off, and she turned another page.

My sister was born at the end of July, 1971. Her birth threw Dorothy into a maelstrom of stress – not postpartum depression, exactly, but something meaner, more vicious, that sank its talons into her mind. According to Slavka, Dad suggested that Dorothy send the baby to live at the Zabrodskys' for a while. I don't think that actually happened. My mother gritted her teeth and clawed her way through the crazy.

"She was really bright, really good for a while. I think she had finally gotten the right dosage of medication. She was doing so well."

Slavka turned one more page. I heard the sigh of her breath over the phone. "Oh, here it is. 'David Zethmayr called me this morning to tell me that Dorothy had fallen and hit her head. She froze to death on the back porch steps.' I was shocked.

"I was one of the first people your dad called. As soon as he told me the news, I was filled with love and sorrow for my sister in Christ. The sisterhood of the church gathered together to plan a nice funeral supper for after the service. Dorothy didn't think she had many friends, because she always kept to herself. But we all came together for her."

My godmother's voice was gentle as she relived the sorrow, more than forty years past. "All I've got are good things to say about her. Nothing bad. I wrote it down in my journal – 'What a simple, trusting child of God.' That was my epitaph for your mom."

I have known my mother dead for far longer than I knew her living. I was five years old, and my sister was two, when our mother slipped and fell on the back porch steps while taking out the garbage on a cold January night.

I remember very little about her – longish dark hair, a mouth that smiled very seldom, a voice that seemed mostly to be yelling ... or crying. My memories of those years consist mostly of scenes, vignettes, snapshots removed from any context.

I do remember a few happy moments in the confusing haze of being a toddler. One that stands out – possibly because Dorothy was in a good mood – is the memory of my mommy showing me a sweet surprise on the kitchen counter: a frosted Easter lamb cake, its head turned to regard me with sugar-dot eyes. I fell in love with that little lamb instantly, and I remember the shock of never seeing it again after that big reveal. (I realize now that two-year-old me was a bit fuzzy on the concept of "edible" – that once you bring a lamb cake to church to share, it's not going to last long. I suppose I should be grateful I didn't see them cutting the cake into pieces. I'd have been scarred for life.)

Other than that, I can't remember my mother being a huge part of my life. She was just there, and I was aware of her the way any five-year-old is aware of anyone. She picked me up from daycare, she took me to ballet class, she turned on the TV for my daily dose of Sesame Street and Zoom, she threatened my father with a brandished frying pan ... the usual.

Then came the morning my father sat us down at the dining room table. He put down three bowls of oatmeal with raisins – one for me, one for my sister, one for himself. My sister and I happily dug in, but my father's oatmeal went untouched. When our spoons clicked on the bottom of the bowls, my dad took a deep breath and probably said something like, "Girls, I have something to tell you..."

I have absolutely no recollection of the next few moments. I have no memory at all of hearing of my mother's death. My memory picks up again several minutes, surely no more than half an hour later. I am standing next to my parents' bed. My mother isn't there. But my father is weeping, and drying his eyes on his white Fruit of the Loom undershirt.

My father was working at Northwestern Hospital, on rotating shifts. That night, he'd been working at the Clinical Chemistry lab. His carpool buddy dropped him off at around 2 am. When Dad didn't find Dorothy in bed, where she should have been at that hour, he probably went through the house, calling for her. Dad found Dorothy unresponsive on the back porch, and carried her into the house to perform CPR on her on the kitchen floor, just inside the back door. But by then it was far too late. If an ambulance came in the small hours of the morning, it arrived with its lights off, its siren silenced. No need to wake the neighbors. If the paramedics pulled up the driveway and wheeled a gurney over the bricks of the back walk to retrieve my mother's body, they did it quietly. I slept through it all.

My grandmother came in from California. Again, I have a fuzzy five-year-old's recollection of the whole situation, but I do remember realizing I was going to spend the summer with my Grandma Ruth, my father's mother. My two-year-old sister, meanwhile, was packed off to stay the summer with my Grandma Marion – Dorothy's mother – when Marion returned to California after the funeral.

Five year olds have a woolly grasp on reality, to say the least. My mother was gone, and it had something to do with that dark brown box I'd seen her lying in at St. Nicholas Church. My father was ... preoccupied. To a little kid, a summer is eternity. I was old enough to realize that this was the most viable option for our fractured little family. I was also young enough to have the glimmer of an idea in my mind that maybe they were taking my sister away from me forever. I knew enough to realize that California was a really, really long ways away, and that's where my sister was going. My world had exploded.

I retreated deeply into the world of books. I taught myself how to read when I was two, and now, reading became even more of an escape. (My sister says her only recollection of being told of our mother's death is intertwined with my experience. When we were both grown, she told me, "When Dad told us that Dorothy was dead, you had just finished reading *Charlotte's Web* for the second time. That's how I processed it – Charlotte died at the end of the book, and so did Dorothy. But I can't remember a thing about being told.")

When I was a teenager, I found a few of Dorothy's journals in our attic, along with the manuscripts of a children's book (about a little duck named Pato) and the rough draft of a short story. The stories were fascinating – I had no idea my mother had dreams, just as I did, of being a writer. The journals, though, were a bit of a letdown. Except for a few mentions of me ("Sylvie and her sister are hiding behind the couch, playing with a broken test-tube ..."), the journals seemed to be little more than laundry lists of the drugs Dorothy was taking, mostly to combat depression. All I knew at that time was that this daily cocktail had led, indirectly, to Dorothy's death.

But a funny thing happened as I was writing this book. Rhoda Derry's story was so compelling to me, even a century later, that I wanted to find a way to bring it even closer to people. I wanted to bring Rhoda's nineteenth century experience forward, to make it a little more relatable. I thought, who do I know that lived through the tumultuous, confusing times of the 1960s? Who struggled with personal demons at the same time society was sending her conflicting messages, the way Rhoda did?

The answer, when it came, was crystal-clear and completely heartbreaking in its simplicity.

I would write about my mother.

I asked my sister, who still visits the house where we grew up, if she had any of our mother's journals.

She did. These were not the journals I read as a teenager. These were journals of Dorothy's I had never seen before – ones she had kept during her childhood in Argentina, that chronicled her move to the United States, to the same house in which her daughters grew up. There was even a journal that included my appearance into the world.

In July of 2013, I made the three hour drive up to Chicago for a family reunion. I stayed at my sister's house, and headed home Sunday afternoon. Nestled in my backpack as I roared down the highway on my black Ducati were four of Dorothy's journals.

I had known my mother dead for most of my life. It was time to meet my mother alive.

As a young woman, Dorothy McClaren was pretty, vivacious, and whip-smart. Her father, Lauren, was an engineer who worked for Armour in one of their meat-packing plants in Argentina. My mother spent her grade-school years, and the first two years of high school, living in wealthy expatriate comfort in Buenos Aires. She was multilingual; she grew up speaking Spanish as much as she did English. She met my father when they were both in German Club in high school. He was a senior and the club president, and she was a junior. Dad was intrigued by anything foreign, and Dorothy had just moved back to the States. She was fiercely intelligent – she had plans, even as she was battling mental illness as an adult, to teach herself Russian and Greek.

She was very pretty, too. My father says when she was younger and in good health, she looked very much like Grace Kelly, about the time of Kelly's marriage to Prince Rainier, around 1959. Personally, I think she bears an uncanny resemblance to the writer Sylvia Plath. I have three pictures of Dorothy, and in one of them she is standing in front of the fireplace in the house where I grew up. She is wearing the blue graduation robes of Lyons Township High School, and she is beaming with pride.

She was tall. Her journals chronicle a constant struggle with her weight, but she was five feet ten inches tall, and not heavy for her height. (My dad, who is six feet tall, asked my sister once, "How did you and Sylvia end up so short?" My sister pointed out that the Bohnhoffs, Dad's parent's generation, were all short folks – his Uncle Bud being the tallest at five feet four inches. His Army papers put him at five feet five inches. The family story goes that when Bud fell short at his physical exam, Bud's superiors told him to come back in the morning to be measured again, because "everyone knows you're taller in the morning after a good night's sleep". In reality, my great-uncle spent the night in the hospital in traction to gain an extra temporary inch for Uncle Sam. For the rest of his life, he couldn't believe his folks bought the "taller in the morning" cover story.)

The journal my mother kept in Argentina, dated 1958, tells the daily life of a happy, carefree sixteen year old girl. She writes of going on vacations, of going to the movies with any one of several boyfriends. (I was deeply pleased to read that one of her beaus, a fellow named Gary, rode a motorcycle. He was one of the guys she seemed pretty serious about, too.)

The journal that begins in Argentina and ends in Illinois is a lovely hard-bound book, the pages marked with the days of the year in Spanish. Inside are the usual preoccupations of a sixteen year old girl – juggling boyfriends, babysitting, reading science fiction novels, going out horseback riding and out for ice cream. Dorothy gets into her fair share of teenage trouble, too. On April 16, she stayed out too late. "Got home at 7:30 & parents were mad as hell ... were ready to call cops."

The family was quite well-off. Dorothy writes about the maid moving her clothes while straightening. In the same entry, she mentions that Janie, her sister, would be entering Radcliffe in the spring. (Janie, also known as Marlys, would later go on to earn a Master's in anthropology from Harvard, and publish many papers and several books on Mayan linguistics. She also had the questionable habit of bringing Indian women home with her when she traveled to South America on her field research trips, and keeping them as poorly-paid housemaids. I guess she wanted to keep up the standard of living she'd gotten used to in Buenos Aires.) The same maid got into trouble when she took off for a vacation and returned several days later than she was supposed to. The family took the opportunity to go into the maid's room, and there they found a lot of their belongings, including a pen with Dorothy's name on it, and a pair of Lauren's underwear. (Dorothy's comment: "Ugh!")

My mother was very pious. Scattered throughout the 1958 diary are notes like, "That which is for our highest good will surely come about. Amen," and "I hope God is still out there watching out for me." She ends each entry with the notation IHS, and explains it once: "I mustn't forget what IHS means. I write it mechanically instead of thinking about it. In His Service. In God's and Jesus' service, Amen." She prays in particular for her father. Lauren McClaren suffered from liver trouble – that seems to be the reason for the family's eventual move back to the States. As Dorothy noted on January 30, "He wants American doctors working on him." Peppered throughout the 1958 journal is the prayer "God please take care of my Daddy."

Dorothy enjoyed school, and she was an excellent student. She commuted by train from a suburb outside the city: Acasuso, or perhaps Bertolome Mitre. She mentions being good at geometry, and getting one hundred percent on a French test – the best score in the class. Her essay "The Responsibility of Parents" was published in the school magazine, Bulletin Board. For this, she got four contributor's copies. Even though she whines, on September 22, "I hate Mondays", that's also the day she was nominated for president of the Spanish Club. (She lost.) And despite her diligence as a student, she can't resist jotting, on June 16, "No more pencils, no more books, no more teachers' dirty looks. If they try to ring the bell, tell them all to go to hell."

But even in the midst of this idyllic late 1950s life, there are signs of trouble. On January 6, she writes at the bottom of the page, "Don't let them know what you're thinking, ever." And again on January 21, at the bottom of the page, in urgent printing instead of her usual teenage cursive, she writes, "Don't get mad and don't tell everything you know."

This could be read as normal teenage angsty paranoia, except for the stories she shared with my father before she died, stories my father later told me when I was old enough to understand them. Darkness was creeping around the corners of her childhood, and she was smart enough to see it, but too young to do anything about it.

There is a throwaway sentence at the end of the entry for January 19, after "Sandy [her dog] ate half a cake": "Daddy killed Teddy Bear's seven kittens (one day old) today. R.I.P." This bare sentence doesn't tell the whole story. Not all abuse is physical, and there was an insidious horror underlying Dorothy's casual "R.I.P.". Her father put the unwanted kittens into a shoebox, along with a rag soaked in chloroform. Then he made Dorothy hold the shoebox lid down, until she could no longer feel the kittens' little heads bumping up against the lid of the box in a frantic search for air.

The end of the 1958 journal tells of the family's trip by boat to San Francisco, then the car trip across country to Illinois, to the house in the Chicago suburbs where I would eventually grow up.

Fast-forward ten years. The bright teenager is gone – it's hard to believe she even existed. She has been replaced by an anxious, fretful, deeply unhappy young woman. During those ten years, Dorothy graduated from high school, met and married my father, and converted from Methodism to the Orthodox faith. My parents suffered the loss of their firstborn child, my brother Stephen, who lived for three days in December 1965 before dying of a hole in his heart. My parents were desperately poor, living in a series of apartments in Chicago, or with my Grandpa Mac and Grandma Marion in the house in the suburbs.

The first half of this journal is bravely hopeful. Dorothy is on mild tranquilizers for her anxiety, not on anything harder, due to her pregnancy with yours truly. She finds comfort in her writing. "The note-book is an entirely previously-unknown level of freedom – no one will jump out of the note-book to tell me I'm no good." She suffers from depression and multiple personality disorder, and she knows it. But she still tries to soldier on in spite of her obvious mental illness issues. She gamely writes reviews of the books she is reading – books like Ernie Pyle's *Brave Men* and the works of Anne Frank and Pearl S. Buck. She still displays a fierce intellect, despite the seriousness of her mental condition. She has moments of chilling lucidity, as when she writes, "I'm not stupid. I know these drugs are going to kill me someday."

Some of the reading sends chills down my spine. On February 25, 1968, when she is three months pregnant with me, she writes, "I just wish I didn't have this 'chick' in my belly ... poor kid. Nobody wants her but her daddy, and she's in her mommy's way in her attempts to stay alive – or dead. What happens when she's here? If there's an accident and she dies, I'll probably land in the nuthouse again. If she lives, how will she grow up and how can I manage?" Her ambivalence and paranoia can be explained, somewhat, by Stephen's death less than three years before. It still gives me the creeps, though.

Three days later, she writes, "Nothing bad today. I believed then that this was all a mistake, and when David came home I asked him I'm not really sick, am I? It was just a mistake. But he said, you are really very sick. I don't feel very sick except I would like *so* terribly much to throw something of glass very hard against the wall and have it break and then maybe cut myself with the glass. When the feeling first came I almost picked up the Vicks Vaporub jar to throw, fascinated by the combination of glass and goo, but then I didn't dare for fear David would hit me or send me to Cook County." I feel a strange combination of terror, sympathy, and admiration whenever I read this. The honesty it took to write this, even in the safety of her journal, is staggering.

March 15, 1968. Dorothy mentions reading *The Three Faces of Eve*. She finds nothing in the book that speaks to her condition, and she dismisses it as "fiction". But then she speaks very frankly about her different personalities, including one she calls The Cat. On April 2 she writes, "The Cat is very interesting. She doesn't like to be addressed by that name ... sometimes when she can't stay any longer she still won't let any other personality take over ... She is very ill-mannered and sneering. She hates authority and enjoys looking challengingly at the one she's talking to with a horrible half-smile, half-sneer on her mouth." (A couple of years later, her therapist would suggest that Dorothy write a book herself, along the lines of *The Three Faces of Eve*. Who knows? If she had had confidence in herself, if her mind could have settled down long enough for her to concentrate, my mother might have written one of the classics of mental health literature. We'll never know.)

One of the most wrenching entries comes on March 27, 1968. It's Lent, and Dorothy is going through yet another dark night of the soul. She pours out a plea to God. I can see an echo of the trusting, childish prayers jotted down in the Argentina notebook, but now there is a grown woman's urgent cry for help. This is the prayer of a drowning, panicking woman.

"God, please find me and love me and never let me go ever. Please forgive me *all* my badnesses and love me and choose me for one of Yours. I love You so, still and always. And I am very puzzled and lost and don't know who to ask about guidance toward You or how not to offend You in my circumstances. Please don't send me to Hell and please let David and me and the baby come to Heaven. Please by Your power come and find me and hear me and cleanse me and forgive me and love me and keep me by You forever. Please, God my Father and Christ my Brother. Please. I don't know where I am – I don't even know who I am or if I am at all. I doubt that I am, so I can't help You find me but you are God and if You do know where I am please find me and forgive me and love me forever and teach me."

Then the baby comes. Dorothy is no longer shackled by the physical limitations of pregnancy, and the prescription drug use begins in earnest. She is almost clinically obsessed with documenting the effects of the sedatives. A typical entry will begin, "Time now is 7:30 pm. At 5 I took four Vistaril, four Noludar, and the third Dilantin, so writing at present is rather difficult." (In one entry, she notes with inebriated solemnity, "It is not advisable to write further at this time.") Then she begins to write. Within two notebook pages, three if she works with fevered ferocity, her handwriting devolves from a looping cursive to an illegible scrawl that meanders for another half a page before the pen finally drops from her numb fingers.

My father tries to help her. When her handwriting trails off, he takes over for her sometimes, chronicling the medication that has just hijacked her fine motor functions. On the page for Easter Sunday, April 13, there is my mother's trailing scribble, followed by a notation in my father's neat, compact, computer programmer's handwriting: "Two Tuinal. God help us."

In the next two journals, from May 14, 1970 to May 15, 1973, Dorothy's world shrinks even farther. The girl who once wrote about exploring the ship that was taking her from Argentina to the United States is now reduced to describing the four walls of her bedroom. Some days it's all she can do to get out of bed and stumble through a day.

"This is a complete, I hope, list of medication prescribed for me at one time or another." The list has forty-one entries, including Quaaludes, barbiturates, tranquilizers, Valium (which she notes as "not effective"), and sodium amytal. Most are sleeping pills, mood elevators, and drugs to combat her debilitating headaches. This last journal I have of my mother's work is the most jarring. In it, she speaks candidly of the thirteen episodes of shock treatment she endured for the treatment of epilepsy. She writes of wishing desperately for some marijuana. She says "fuck".

Dorothy's journal entry for July 16, 1971, just a couple of weeks before my sister was born, has words I never expected to hear from either one of my parents: "I'd sure like to smoke some marijuana." Later that night, in an entry labeled midnight, Dorothy's wry sense of humor tries to reassert itself.

"Well, what do you know! Something I had been wondering upon, lo these many months [of being pregnant]. I'm still a drug addict." She writes of her physical and mental reaction to taking a mild sleeping pill safe to take towards the end of pregnancy. That mild dose gave her a much-missed sense of euphoria.

"I learned several things while it was 'on' – one being that I would jeopardize myself and my family for more more more ... Yes, I would go back on [drugs] instantly if I could figure out where to get what." I had never read a *cri de coeur* quite like that. I certainly never expected to read it in my mother's journal.

The next day is even worse. Whatever my mother had been running from had finally caught her. It knocked her down, and now it was sitting on her and howling hot breath in her face. Dorothy took two more sleeping pills. Using her journal as an outlet for her guilt (or lack of it), she snarls, "No point in asking me what about the baby – how the hell do I know 'what about the baby'?"

About forty-five minutes after taking the first pill, Dorothy cuts herself with a razor blade, four slices on her wrist. "Not serious enough to need stitches – after all, I didn't have suicide in mind. So why did I do it at all? I don't know. No little voice told me to. I just wanted to ... I don't feel remorseful or repentant, not even my usual terror of God's anger ... I just feel a mixture of nothing and of screaming frustration – I must have more drugs! Now! And how and where can I get the fuckin' things ... Sylvia saw the gauze I had wrapped around my wrist. I told her it was a bandage 'cause I hurt myself. Oh, oh oh oh God I must have some drugs." It's a stressed-out lament, a plea for relief from the hamster wheel of anxieties her mind had become.

Every summer, my aunt Mary Lu hosts a family reunion at the old homestead in the Chicago suburbs, the house my Grandpa Gordon built – the house where I did a lot of my growing up. Whenever I'm there, it's hard for me to realize that when the visit is over, I have to get in the car and drive for three hours to get home ... I feel like I'm home already. My aunt Karen and her husband come down from Wisconsin, and so do my cousins. My cousin Hilary often flies in from San Francisco. It's an excuse to get together on a summer weekend and enjoy food, music (we're a family of musicians), and reminiscing over family stories. That weekend gives us a chance to reforge our roots by sharing the well-worn memories of family members who've gone before us.

We have no shortage of funny, interesting, sometimes embarrassing stories about our forebears. Aunt Marj (my grandmother's sister) was an expert fencer in high school, who would have gone to the Olympics if they hadn't been held in Berlin that year – the year being 1936. Marj worked in the microbiology lab at the University of Chicago, and discovered several strains of venereal disease. She also didn't suffer fools gladly – or at all. One day one of the other scientists sidled up to Marj where she was working at a lab station, and tried to slide a hand up her skirt. She whirled around, snatched a couple of bills from her pocket, threw them at him, and snarled, "Here's two bucks – go get yourself a whore."

Marj never married, preferring instead to live with her parents, Edwin and Anna Bohnhoff. Grandpa Bohnhoff, after he retired, swore he would never again get out of bed before nine in the morning. At 8:48 one chilly morning, the electric blanket he was using began to smolder. Grandpa just lay there, slitting his eyes against the growing haze of smoke. The blanket burst into flame right at nine am, and that's when Grandpa hopped out of bed and smothered the fire.

On the other side of the family, Great-grandma Margaret was an endless fount of the bizarre. She fancied herself a poet, and wrote incessantly. When she picked up a pen, no surface was safe. She wrote on photographs, tables, desks, even pillar candles. Aunt Mary Lu has a cup and saucer that still bore traces of Margaret's scribbling up until a few years ago, when a housekeeper accidentally washed it. Our family history is rich with storytelling, in any medium.

In 2015, while I was working on this book, Camp Zethmayr was held in August. Various combinations of aunts, uncles, siblings, and cousins gathered on the deck outside the back door, the groups constantly shifting as people left to refill plates, or came back out with glasses of sangria or lemonade. I finished the last bite of my brownie, and looked around at the family members sitting there – my father among them. Now, I decided, was as good a time as any.

"Hey, you know how we always tell Grandma Ruth stories, and Grandpa Gordon stories, and Aunt Marj stories? We even tell crazy Grandma Margaret stories ... but we never tell Dorothy stories. Why is that?"

I had the sense that I was picking up a thick stick to bash in a hornet's nest, but the words were out of my mouth before I could stop them, hanging in the air like a fart after my sister's famous family-reunion taco bar. My uncle Jim, the only family member there besides my father who would have remembered Dorothy, looked vaguely uncomfortable. His wife, my aunt Mary Lu, who came into the family years after Dorothy's death, had a look of polite inquiry on her face as she turned towards my dad.

My father sat rigid in his lawn chair. Slowly, carefully, he set his empty plate on the picnic table.

"You want to hear a Dorothy story? Fine." His teeth weren't clenched, exactly, but his tone was clipped and short. "I'll tell you a Dorothy story."

And then he related a story I had read in one of Dorothy's journals. Hearing the incident from a different point of view was strange, and more than a little eerie, like watching a film clip of a car accident from a different angle.

I had come home late from classes one night. Dorothy was already in bed, asleep because she had taken her medication. I went to bed and fell asleep pretty quickly.

Sometime during the night, I woke up suddenly. Dorothy was kneeling next to me – and she was holding a knife to my throat. She had multiple personalities, and one of them was called the Cat. The Cat was evil, and really wanted to kill me. I spoke to Dorothy calmly, trying to get her back. She finally came back to herself, and I rolled over and went back to sleep.

"There you go. There's a Dorothy story for you." My father stood abruptly and stalked off of the deck and down into the back yard. The rest of us sat there, poleaxed. My cousin Hilary was the first to break the brittle silence.

"I think it's natural for you to want to know more about your mother, Sylvie. I don't blame you a bit."

I nodded, still stunned. My aunt shifted in her chair. The pall of my father's story lingered for a few minutes more, as we all digested the slice of horror we'd been served as the dessert to our picnic – at my request.

About five minutes later, my father came back up on the deck. "I figured I shouldn't just leave you with that," he said stiffly. "There were good times too." And he told two stories. Dorothy had a beautiful soprano voice, and Dad said he remembered best two things that made her proud and happy. They happened at Holy Trinity Cathedral, Chicago.

During Great Lent, at a Liturgy of Presanctified, choir director Boris Nikoloff beckoned her and me to step out from the choir with him. Father Madison was facing the altar, ready to intone the refrain to "Let my prayer arise in thy sight as incense and let the lifting up of my hands be an evening sacrifice".

Boris had us stand right behind the priest. He was holding some music for the three of us. Neither Dorothy nor I had ever sung nor seen this setting of the hymn, an STB trio. Boris was perhaps assuming we knew it, or else trusting we could sight-sing it. It went off perfectly. Dorothy and I were both proud of her.

Every week, after Saturday vespers, Father Madison hosted the university kids in his apartment. That Easter, the bunch was gathered around his dining room table singing all the versions of "Xristos voskrese iz smertvi" ("Christ is Risen From the Dead") we could think of.

Among the revelers was a Russian girl with a famously beautiful voice. I could feel Dorothy shrinking into herself as everyone enjoyed Mary's singing.

The group ran out of different musical versions to sing, so Father Hilary started up in Greek: "Xristos anesti ek nekron", and Dorothy and I were the only ones to sing along. That made her proud and happy too.

"April 3, 1968 – Dorothy is bad. She must be punished. How should we punish her? We must punish her soon before she gets away from us."

The Cat was just one of my mother's personalities, but it was easily the most vicious. My mother usually wrote about the Cat after the personality had made her appearance and then left.

So far, these are obviously the deranged scribblings of one of her personalities. Interestingly, the handwriting, although recognizably Dorothy's, is neater and more legible than her usual script. But then, on April 18, halfway through her pregnancy with me, Dorothy writes an entry referring to herself in the third person, writing as if from the viewpoint of one of her alternate personalities. These five pages show her grasp of her situation as much as the entire rest of the journal put together.

The words are flat, calculated, and utterly chilling, completely unlike the hesitant pain of the rest of the journal. My stomach clenched as I read the words. I had been given a rare privilege, something many writers dream of – a look directly into the mind of the person about whom I was writing. But soon, I began to wonder if I really wanted to look into that abyss. I could feel my mother looking dispassionately over my shoulder as I read, watching the back of my neck with cold eyes.

"Dorothy must not be allowed to reach these things. She is a worthless good-for-nothing and she's bad and wicked besides. It is time to put the breaks [sic] on and start the attack. She will probably lose her husband but that is her fault for caring about him and thinking about love, as if she were *people.* I've got the knife hidden away, it remains only to figure out how to use it. I have to scare her though, because she is talking too much ... I don't know who I am, tho' I pretty well know somewhat of who she is. But sometimes she helps me, and I don't know if this is by accident or because she is part me or us. She can't and mustn't go to the hospital, which means the baby's got to go, which means she must be killed. It is too late to kill the baby without pain and fear ... If she lets it be born and then kills it that's her worry. I can't help her there. I suppose she will, tho', because I think she, and we, are all insane. Her husband thinks he helps by telling her to grow up and stop being a child, but it is not the perverse spoiledness of a child that is wrong with her ... And if I keep my end up she'll be so bad off by the time September comes that she'll refuse to go to the hospital, if she hasn't given me a chance to kill the baby and/or her yet. And if she goes to the hospital, I can see from the inside of her that she hasn't got a chance. I don't care, and neither does she. She has moments of thinking she got an unfair deal but on the whole she is convinced of her own shittiness and doesn't want to go on living and have and raise a baby. She truly loves David and he's a marvelous guy but she had no business letting him care for a persona non grata like she is ... David is the only one who could screw up the plans. He might try, tho' I don't see why he thinks it's worth it. Sure she loves him very much but she's extremely ill and he is a very desirable and sweet husband and could find anyone good who isn't sick to marry ... I don't think anyone could ever love him as much as she does but insanity is such a selfish thing ... Poor guy. If only he could see what she needs. But probably it's beyond all human comprehension and ability. He's only human. His tactics of love and kindness as a cure is [sic] very good but humanly he can't help anger and self-condemnation and scolding. Just like a surgeon who takes the risks by opening up an abdomen to cure the patient will lose the patient to infection if he gets impatient or careless and allows the wound to become unsterile, so when David tries this excellent but risky technique of love he should realize that the very procedure which could save her makes her very vulnerable ... He is tired and unsure of himself *because she by the nature of her illness* changes frequently and he interprets these momentary changes to having lost and therefore of being of no worth himself. This of course is as wrong as he could ever be but she can't always pull out of her 'tailspin' soon enough to reassure him. He chose a hard job ... No, Dorothy and all of us have been too ruined and contaminated by her mother and sister ... we cannot escape it and be uncursed and clean."

It was in the September 30 journal entry, written a month after I was born, that Dorothy seems to have had a breakthrough.

The knowledge doesn't seem to have helped her mental state any, because it was after this that she really started hitting the prescription drugs hard. But she came to the realization that most of her mental illness stemmed from a deeply flawed and dysfunctional relationship with her father. Lauren, in turn, was messed up by "frigid Protestant" Marion Green (my grandmother). The relationship between the four of them – Lauren, Marion, Marlys, and Dorothy – was a frozen pond; brittle politeness on the surface, with dark muddy tangles of weeds underneath, ready to pull an unwary swimmer to her breathless doom. Marlys, the older daughter, and Marion were as thick as thieves. Dorothy, the younger, was a "daddy's girl". She sought her mother's attention, but could never get it. There was, I think, some real hatred there, on both sides. And Dorothy suffered her older sister's bullying. As an adult, she told my father that one of Marlys' favorite games was to make Dorothy stand on the garden hose, which Marlys would then yank out from under her feet, dumping Dorothy to the ground. Dorothy fell for this mean trick about as often as Charlie Brown fell for Lucy's football antics.

There were two factions in that family: Mother and Father. And the two daughters chose sides, and ended up not as allies, but as bitter enemies. For someone as naturally sweet as Dorothy was, this must have been a daily hell. The constant stress of keeping up appearances must have been brutal.

What is to be gained by reading these journals? What do I possibly hope to learn by poring over the scribblings of a diseased mind?

My sister and I have very different ways of looking at our mother's journals – as we do about nearly everything.

My sister reads Dorothy's journals with a sense of frustration. "I want to reach through time and just shake her, and say come on, be a parent! Be my mother! Impart some wisdom to me through your words. Stop doctor-hopping, and make better choices, for God's sake. Set attainable goals and hold yourself accountable for them."

My sister shook her head as we talked. She was only two years old when Dorothy died, so she has even fewer memories of our mother than I do. "Mostly I want to ask her, what about you made your mind snap like that?"

A lot of it seems to stem from Dorothy's childhood. Not all abuse is physical, and my mother grew up in a profoundly dysfunctional family. She later had the presence of mind to examine her background from the safety of her journals. The emotional abuse she suffered through was horrific.

My mother grew up desperate to be wanted, to be loved. To be cherished was a goal beyond her wildest aspirations. She would have settled for simple acceptance.

My aunt Karen went to school with Dorothy, her future sister-in-law. She remembers that one day, Dorothy stopped her in the hallway at Lyons Township High School. Dorothy wanted to ask Karen's opinion on taking an advanced psychology class. (Looking back on it, Karen thinks this was one of Dorothy's earliest attempts at trying to figure out what was going on inside her own mind.) During the conversation, Dorothy thrust a picture of her sister Marlys at Karen.

"Isn't she pretty?" Dorothy asked, almost demanded.

"Well, yes, but you're pretty too," Karen replied.

My sister's attitude towards our mother is mostly one of disappointment. "I want to say, go back to the person you were a few pages ago – sly, facile with language, almost cosmopolitan. I could see there were a couple of times where she got a couple of good ones in at Dad's expense."

It's true. When she was lucid, our mother was talented, witty, and very smart. Every once in a while, her journals reveal brief glimpses of a very likeable person. I like to think I would have gotten along with her, as an adult. In her 1958 journal, the one she kept in Argentina, she mentions events that later showed up in the history books – Alaska joining the union as the 49th state on July 1, and the death of Pope Pius XII on October 8. Her journal entry for February 2 even begins, "History is being made this week: America launched the satellite 'Uncle Sam', and Egypt and Syria are going to form the United Arab Republic." February 6 brought more news: "Sputnik II is circling, rivaled by 'Jupiter Explorer'. The Navy sent one up but it goofed. Scientists talking every day about 'space travel'."

And on December 1, there is the following somber journal entry: "Terrible fire in Our Lady of the Angels, a Catholic school in Chicago. Almost ninety people (eighty-three grade school kids and three nuns) killed and over a hundred injured. Worst school fire in the history of Chicago. Maybe cause [sic] by cigarette, maybe arson."

Dorothy was a smart kid, who grew up to be a smart adult. But she was flawed. My sister and I have had several discussions about what made our father choose Dorothy as a wife. It's possible that he just picked a woman who needed saving – a woman who was so damaged, it didn't matter what kind of personality she had.

To be fair, my sister has more of a reason to be disappointed in our mother than I do. She suffers from prosopagnosia, which is an inability to recognize faces. (If she's watching a movie, and a character is wearing a hat, and is hatless in the next scene, my sister is lost – she has no idea if it's the same actor or not.) The condition has several causes, one of which seems to be neglect at a crucial time in an infant's development. As my parents' second child, my sister drew the short end of the stick when it came to getting attention. I remember my father being very attentive toward my development. I clearly remember being carried on his shoulders as we went for a walk in the yard the evening he taught me to count past one hundred, and the "light bulb moment" that gave me. But by the time my sister came along, Dad was deeply enmeshed in his wife's mental illness. He didn't have the time to devote to my infant sister's cognitive needs the way he did mine.

And my reaction to reading Dorothy's journals?

I devoured 1958. I was tickled to learn that my mother dated a guy who rode a motorcycle – a Ducati, no less. But I slowed down after that. Her journals from 1968 onward are tough going. It's hard to read someone's most personal thoughts, even if they've been dead for decades. It's especially wrenching to read things like: "I have decided to try to get well ... for [Sylvia's] sake. I don't want her, yet I refuse to give up the child of my body, and I can't kill her unless God is merciful and gives me an accident or kills her like Stephen, which I doubt, so I have to get better to take care of her."

On my mother's death certificate, the cause of death is listed as "Noludar intoxication, associated hypothermic exposure". Although there was an autopsy, according to the paperwork, no mention is made of the head injury Dorothy suffered as a result of hitting her head on the steps when she slipped and fell. The blame for her death is laid squarely on the Noludar, and on the freezing cold that in her drugged condition, Dorothy couldn't escape. Noludar has a biological half-life of between six and sixteen hours – plenty of time for a woman to freeze to death while under the soporific influence of the drug.

There is a photograph of my mother, sent to me by my godmother Slavka, that sits in my dining room. The snapshot shows Dorothy, wearing her sheepskin coat, holding my infant sister and beaming at the camera. The date on the back of the photo is November 13, 1971. I remember the muted-leather smell of that coat. I remember burying my face in it on cold winter nights when my mother would carry me in from the car after a visit to my grandmother's house.

Can you miss someone you've never really known? Can you look at a photograph of a parent, taken when she was two decades younger than you are now, and see some of yourself in her face?

Or is it just the idea of "mother" that I miss?

My mother suffered terribly with mental illness for most of her short life. She struggled with anxiety, epilepsy, self-mutilation ... many of the same issues that plagued Rhoda Derry.

If Rhoda's doctors and caretakers had had access to the kinds of medication my mother took for years ... would Rhoda's life have turned out differently? It's a question I haven't yet answered for myself. I may never be able to answer it.

All I know for sure is that Rhoda managed to survive when her brain was trying to kill her. Even with all her paranoia of witchcraft, her depression, her despondency over losing Charles, her self-abuse, being locked up for decades ... Rhoda survived.

My mother was not so lucky.

PART FOUR: RHODA IN THE TWENTY-FIRST CENTURY

CHAPTER-TWENTY TWO
REALITY'S END FILMS

Rhoda hesitated behind the concealing cover of the trunk of the elm tree, thoughtfully bouncing the smooth oval stone in her palm. Should she skip the rock? It was perfect ... but it might not catch his attention. Better just to make a splash. She closed her eyes and took a deep breath, trying to calm her racing heart. He was so very handsome! *Please, please let him talk to me ...*

She stepped out from behind the tree. Here, on the shore of the lake, she could see the ripples in the water as the boy floated, moving his hands in lazy strokes to keep himself floating steady. She caught her lower lip between her teeth as sunlit drops sparkled on his perfect shoulders. *Oh my ...* Before her nerve failed her, she tossed the rock into the water.

It made a loudly satisfying splash, and the boy whipped his head around to see who was interrupting his swim, his wet hair flinging drops of water. His look of confusion softened to a grin when he saw the pretty dark-haired girl on the shore.

"Who are you? Are you a thief?" he teased.

Rhoda tossed her head, indignant. "No, I'm not a thief! I was picking apples, and I ... saw you in the lake." She silently congratulated herself for bringing a basket and a few apples with her. The nearest apple tree was at the far end of her own backyard, and that was a good half-mile walk from the lake. What he didn't know wouldn't hurt him, though.

With a faked sniff of disdain, Rhoda turned and took a few steps away. From the lake, she heard a splash as the boy floundered to stand up. "Wait! Don't go, I want to talk to you. What's your name?"

She smiled to herself. That was better. She pasted a polite smile – her "Sunday best" smile – on her face as she turned.

"I'm Rhoda Derry." Color rose to her cheeks as the boy scrambled, dripping, onto the shore. "Why, you are nearly naked! Do you always swim naked?"

The boy grinned. "Is there another way? Do you swim with your clothes on?"

Rhoda lifted a hand to her burning cheek. "I don't know how to swim." Desperate to change the subject, she blurted, "What's your name, handsome?"

"Charles. Charles Phenix. Don't be afraid – I'll teach you how to swim," he said, reaching for her hand.

Rhoda felt temptation do a joyful leap in her heart as the boy's cool hand closed over hers. As he tugged her closer to the water, though, reason returned.

"It is late and nearly suppertime. My family will be looking for me." Reluctantly, she slipped her hand from Charles', her fingers still tingling from his touch.

"Will I see you again?" Charles called after her.

She threw him a flirty little smile over her shoulder as she walked away.

"If you are lucky."

The Rhoda that appears in the Reality's End film, *The Mysterious Rhoda Derry* is probably more forward than the historical Rhoda. The scriptwriter took a few liberties with Rhoda's story, such as how she and Charles met, in order to tell his version of her tale. Brandon Lamprecht is the writer, director, and producer responsible for bringing Rhoda to life for the Reality's End Films project. Brandon and his crew have put their own interpretive spin on Rhoda's story.

For all the people who've seen the movie trailer on YouTube, April Cowgur is the face of Rhoda Derry. Tall, with long hair the color of the prairie sky on a moonless night, a sweetly smiling mouth, and the dark exotic eyes of an Arabian Nights princess, April is the perfect choice to play the farmer's daughter who captured the heart of Charles Phenix.

April was one of seventy or so girls who answered Reality's End Films' casting call to play the part of Rhoda Derry. Her fiancé, Patrick Thornton, was cast as Charles.

I tried to ask April about her reaction to getting cast as Rhoda, and her feelings about playing such a complex character.

"It was a great experience to film," was her only response. The rest of my Facebook messages, before and after this terse reply, went unremarked and unanswered.

April's reticence to talk about her work on *The Mysterious Rhoda Derry* may stem from the fact that the project was plagued, almost from the beginning, with setbacks. And I'm not talking about actors flubbing their lines, or the crew showing up late for a shoot. I'm talking straight-up *Twilight Zone: The Movie* weirdness. Strange accidents. The brakes going out on Brandon's car. Unexplained illnesses. One of the more experienced stunt riders took a nasty tumble off his horse for no discernable reason. He was fine, and kept on filming the next day. But the crew was still shaken up.

And the unsettling occurrences weren't limited to happenings on the set. While the actors and crew were in the middle of filming, someone called in a bomb threat to the preschool where Brandon's child was a student at the time.

"It was in Tremont! You know what a small town Tremont is. Who calls in a bomb threat to a *preschool*? In *Tremont*?" Brandon's voice was thick with disbelief when he told me about it.

"It started off very subtle. Glasses falling off a counter for no reason and breaking. Seeing things out of the corner of your eye that can be brushed off as nothing. We didn't even realize something was going on until the really bad stuff started happening. Then we started to put the pieces together."

Brandon shies away from too much discussion of the misfortunes that have followed the filming of *The Mysterious Rhoda Derry*. He will say that NAMI heard about the project and contacted him, but even with their interest, Reality's End decided to stop work on the film. Brandon gets questions all the time, even some from paranormal investigators, asking if Rhoda has somehow cursed the project.

"It always seems to happen around Halloween," Brandon says. "I'm just afraid that hers is a tale remembered for ghoulish pleasure to satisfy fans of the supernatural. Upon scrolling through some comments on our documentary, I realized many people just wanted to see a crazy story about a woman in a box who removed her eyes." Possible paranormal weirdness aside, Brandon has no wish to tell Rhoda's story solely for the sake of perpetuating the gruesome details of her life.

Reality's End Films has suspended work on *The Mysterious Rhoda Derry*. As of this writing, the project is on indefinite hold. Brandon has been spooked by the strange experiences that have plagued the production, and he doesn't want to encourage the myth of the Curse of Rhoda Derry.

Those who want to get a taste of the project, though, are free to visit YouTube. There are a few scenes available, as well as a short teaser for the film.

As they were filming, Brandon kept a secret. No one – not the actors, not Brandon's film crew, not the historical advisors – not one of them knew of the deep connection he felt for Rhoda. Not one of them knew how very personal Rhoda's story was for Brandon.

CHAPTER TWENTY-THREE
PARALLEL LIVES

Once upon a time, there was a boy who loved a girl. They were teenagers, but each knew they'd found their soulmate.

The boy's family was well-off – not rich, but comfortable. The girl's family, not so much. The girl's father worked hard for a living, but ends never really seemed to meet unless they stretched an awfully long way.

But that didn't matter to the young couple. Money didn't matter, feuding families didn't matter – not as long as they had each other. The only thing that mattered was their love. They even talked about getting married one day.

All of that changed, though, when the boy was forbidden to see the girl. The girl, distraught at the loss of her love, began to self-harm, and was eventually committed to an asylum.

If this sounds familiar to you, you're right. It's Rhoda's story.

It's also Brandon Lamprecht's story.

When Brandon was a teenager, he fell in love. His girlfriend was the daughter of a guy who worked at Caterpillar, the big equipment manufacturing company based in Peoria. Brandon's dad was a Cat executive.

In the early 1990s, Caterpillar workers went on strike. It was a big deal, as Cat is one of the largest employers in the Peoria area.

One of the casualties of the strike was Brandon's relationship. The girlfriend's father went on strike against Brandon's father. Things got messy, and Brandon was forbidden to see his girlfriend.

Devastated, Brandon threw himself into his filmmaking. He buried himself in his work, taking on project after project, trying to outrun the heartache. And every one of them, he worked on with his girlfriend in mind.

He heard through the grapevine that his girlfriend had tried to harm herself. She had been committed to a psych ward. Physically, she was okay, but she was grieving Brandon's loss. There was nothing he could do for her, or for himself.

He'd been ordered by his father to keep his distance. So he kept on working, making films, and dedicating each project to her.

In 2010, Reality's End Films made a film called *The Asylum Chronicles 1: Bookbinder*. The film tells the story of one of the patients at the Peoria State Hospital, a man whose ghost showed up at his own funeral. The period piece got good reviews, and has been shown to sold-out crowds at local theaters. It has been aired on fifty-seven different public access channels in Illinois, from the Chicago suburbs to Springfield, and you can find it on YouTube.

But Brandon wasn't finished telling tales of the Peoria State Hospital – not yet. Soon after filming *Bookbinder*, Brandon learned of another patient at the asylum.

He heard the story of Rhoda Derry.

Brandon was rocked to his core at the similarities between Rhoda's story and his own life. He knew that Reality's End Films had to tell Rhoda's tale. They began filming, and no one knew that as Brandon was telling the story of Rhoda and Charles, he was also honoring his own tale of love and loss. April Cowgur was cast as Rhoda mostly because of her resemblance to Brandon's girlfriend. And the music in one of the movie trailers – U2's "With or Without You" – that's their song.

A few years ago, Brandon's girlfriend came out of seclusion. She contacted him. In the years since they'd last seen each other, Brandon had gotten married, and divorced. They both had to wonder: were the feelings still there?

They were. Brandon and his girlfriend are still soulmates. They are taking things slow for now, but the future looks bright with possibility. They may start dating again. In July 2016, Brandon changed his Facebook status to a simple "In a relationship". No details, just those three simple words.

Maybe this time around, the story will have a happy ending.

CHAPTER TWENTY-FOUR
RHODA'S FAMILY

D. Doc Derry is descended from Basil and Fredericka Derry. He grew up hearing stories of his great-aunt Rhoda, stories passed down through the years, of Rhoda spinning on her head like a top, or Rachel shooting at imaginary witches in the house. These stories fired his imagination as a child. When he grew up, he channeled that fascination with history into the study of the genealogy of the Derry family and its branches. He has written a book about the Derry family's most famous member. Doc's book, *Rhoda: A Tragic and True Story of a Farmer's Daughter*, is a love letter to his great-aunt.

Doc is a grey-haired bear of a man, whose voice on the phone perfectly matches his pictures on Facebook. He is devoted to keeping alive the memories of those who have gone before him.

"I do believe Jacob and Rachel had a good family life ... though poor, it was a close family while Jacob and Rachel were alive. When the two oldest sons moved from Indiana to the Quincy area, it wasn't long before the rest of the family followed."

His voice is a gentle rumble as he talks about Rhoda. "According to all accounts, Rhoda was a beautiful young woman during her teen years, even into her early twenties. That's how I like to remember her."

I met Chad Derry when he came out to Bartonville to visit the grave of his famous relative. Chad is related to Rhoda, but not quite as closely as Doc is. Chad Derry is a distant cousin of both Doc and Rhoda. The two Derry family lines diverged in the early 1700s, between Doc's third great-grandfather Valentine Derry and Chad's sixth great-grandfather Peter Derry. But Chad has a soft spot for his long-lost relative and her story.

We met at Rhoda's grave, and talked about her tragic history, and her eventual rescue by Dr. Zeller. I filled in some details for Chad, things about Rhoda – and Old Moll – that he hadn't heard yet. For my part, I was thrilled to meet another of Rhoda's relatives.

Chad had been to the Peoria State Hospital before, and had gone on an investigation in the Bowen Building. He described for me a ghost photograph he had snapped – a misty shape down a hallway that he very much hoped was Rhoda. (Actually, Rhoda never set foot in the Bowen Building, but the photograph may very well show someone else – a nurse, perhaps.)

We walked back to our vehicles after visiting Rhoda's grave ~ I to my Mustang, he to his red pickup truck. As I put my hand on the door handle, Chad fixed me with a serious look. "I want you to put something in that book you're writing."

Something in the look on his face made me pause, and I walked back to him. "Yeah? What's up?"

His eyes were shaded by the brim of his ball cap as he spoke. "Make sure you tell people that the Derrys are just regular, ordinary folks. We're not a bunch of evil wizards and witches."

Then a grin broke across his face. "Except for my ex-wife ... but she's not really a Derry, so I don't guess she counts."

CHAPTER TWENTY-FIVE
RHODA'S SPIRIT

When it comes to the paranormal, the Peoria State Hospital is an extremely active site. The history of the place, with its legacy of care and compassion, contributes to the hauntings on the hilltop. The spirits are there not because they are trapped in misery, but because they have returned to a place where they felt loved.

Rhoda seems to be one of those spirits. Peoria State Hospital lore says Rhoda loved the entire hilltop so much, her spirit can be felt anywhere up there. But the strongest chance a visitor has to experience her ghost is when they're standing at Rhoda's grave in Cemetery One. Rhoda never lost the habit of chewing tobacco, the habit she'd picked up as a teenager. When she lived at the asylum, she still enjoyed a plug now and then. If she knew a visitor had some tobacco in his pocket, she would crab across the floor and tug on his pants leg to request a chaw. It's said that when you're standing at the gravesite, if you smell chewing tobacco, and feel a gentle tugging on your pants leg, that's Rhoda trying to get your attention.

One night I was hanging out with a group of ghost hunters at the Pollak Hospital, the former TB ward on the hilltop. We were in the Women's Ward, and the energy that night was rather low ... there just wasn't much going on. To pass the time, I told the group the story of Rhoda Derry. After the tale was told, we all decided to make our way back to the front of the building.

As we left the Women's Ward, every single one of us smelled the distinctive odor of chewing tobacco.

James Barrow is a ghost hunter who has a passion for the Peoria State Hospital. He explores the grounds and the buildings every chance he gets. Long ago, he got into the habit of letting his voice recorder run as he walked around the grounds. Happily for James, Rhoda has gotten to know him through his many visits to the asylum ... and she has a soft spot for him.

Several years ago, James was visiting Rhoda's grave, and he happened to remark to another investigator that he had meant to bring some tobacco for Rhoda as a gift. Moments later, a gravelly voice showed up on James' recorder.

The voice said, *"That's okay ... I can't chew anymore."*

Another time, James had gone to the Pollak Hospital's Haunted Infirmary attraction, held every Friday and Saturday night in October. After the haunt closed for the night, James strolled down the block to Cemetery One to visit Rhoda. Of course, he had his recorder going. When reviewing the recording later, he heard a woman's voice say, *"James, come on down and sit."* Now, this voice may not have been Rhoda. But she is so fond of James, that it is possible that Rhoda was inviting him to "set a spell" on a brisk October night.

James emailed me yet another story. "I had a run in with her on December 6 while alone on the second floor of the Bowen. I had just come from a truly frightening experience at Springdale Cemetery [in Peoria] so I was quite jittery. Around the middle of the main corridor I happened to feel a sharp and quite noticeable tug on my left pants leg, and I asked Rhoda if that was her. I didn't hear a response then, but when I played my recorder when I got home, I heard a faint *"It's Rhoda Derry"* before I asked my question. It was followed by a man's and a child's voice, and then Rhoda piped up again saying *"I need a chew"*." (I'd like to point out that it's unusual to encounter Rhoda in the Bowen Building, as she was never within its walls in life. But Rhoda seems to be attracted to James. Is it possible she ventured into the building just to visit with him?)

There is one more personal experience that someone shared with me that seems to involve Rhoda Derry. Once more, it's odd, because it took place in the Bowen Building.

"I was investigating in the basement," Jamee Congrove told me, "and we were in the small room at the end of the hallway nearest Pfeiffer Road, the room they call the chapel." I nodded. "The chapel" is a flight of fancy, but the room is beautiful, with a fireplace and a mantelpiece of greenish marble.

"I was in the room, looking around, and I saw a shadow figure crouched on the floor. It wasn't just short, like a child's spirit might be, it was definitely taller but crouched, you know, hunched over. And it scuttled on all fours. It scrabbled towards me, then vanished. But I think that was Rhoda."

There were sixty-three buildings on the hilltop at the asylum's height. Twelve of those buildings are left. The C Row cottage in which Rhoda spent the last two years of her life is long gone. But Dining Hall A, where Rhoda was moved after her diagnosis, and where she passed away on October 9, 1906, still stands.

Dining Hall A is a pleasantly unassuming one-story building, a compact place of light brown brick with neat stone accents at each corner. Every window – and there are many windows, on every side of the building – is topped with a precise arch of brick. Light pours in through the tall windows. It is a calm, beautiful place to sit and enjoy the fellowship of a meal.

It is also, I imagine, a calm, beautiful place to spend one's last few months of life.

I wanted desperately to get into Dining Hall A while working on this book. What better place to try to contact Rhoda's spirit than the building in which she passed away? Unfortunately, circumstances dictated that as of the time this book went to press, a paranormal investigation of the building was quite impossible.

But as things turned out, I didn't need to get into Dining Hall A to experience an encounter with Rhoda.

In early July 2016, Shadow Hunters, led by Nick Sarlo, came to the Pollak Hospital for two solid nights of investigation. They were joined by Archer Paranormal Investigations, out of Georgia, and the Florida-based group ESP – Explorers of Spirit Phenomena.

The members of all three groups were relaxed, but completely professional as they wandered the halls of the hospital with their equipment. I was able to tag along with them both Friday and Saturday nights.

The experience was astounding. I've been at the Pollak many times, and I have never seen it as active as I did that weekend. We captured EVPs, we saw things move by themselves – it was astonishing.

Not all of the groups' experiences were so dramatic. Some were intensely personal. Two of the ladies that joined us that weekend had psychic encounters with Rhoda.

Liz Nygard, of Shadow Hunters, and Lisa Shackelford, the lead investigator of Archer Paranormal, agree that on the Other Side, Rhoda looks very different from the emaciated wreck in her photograph. Liz is empathic, and there is a powerful genetic component to her abilities. Many women in her family, including her grandmother and great-grandmother, are sensitive to psychic energy. Liz says with a grin, "I'm basically a walking sonar dish."

Liz was deeply affected by Rhoda's story, so much so that she would not use her name in casual conversation with me. She preferred instead to say "girlfriend down there in the cemetery", or "your girl". Liz assured me Rhoda has returned to the physical appearance in which she feels most comfortable.

"If you see a proper Victorian lady on the grounds of the asylum, and you can't quite place her ... ask her what her name is," Liz offered.

Lisa had her own encounter with Rhoda's spirit. On Friday night, all of the investigators split up into small groups to explore the hospital. The group I was with gravitated to the Women's Ward, while Lisa's group spent some time in the doll room. Lisa was standing in the room when she felt hands grasping her leg, below the knee. She spoke up and reported it to the group. One of the guides said, "That could be Rhoda."

"I got chills up and down my spine when she said that." Lisa describes herself as an intuitive medium. She has an experiment that she does to test the validity of the experiences she has. She uses the intuitive power of her own body, acting as a human-sized pendulum to gauge the truth. She will stand up straight and say, "In Divine Truth, do I like chocolate?" Her body will tilt forward in a positive answer. She'll reset herself, standing straight once again: "In Divine Truth, is my hair black and curly?" A negative answer will cause her body to tilt backward. She'll get an "icky, sinky" feeling, and her shoulders will hunch as her body reacts negatively. After an unseen entity clasped her leg, Lisa tested the guide's theory. "In Divine Truth, did I have an experience with Rhoda Derry?"

Her body dipped forward with the truth.

All the rest of that evening, and for the next afternoon, Lisa thought about the encounter.

"I thought, gosh, it's so unfair that even after all she suffered in life, in the afterlife she's still crawling on the floor."

But early on Saturday evening, Lisa's psychic talents showed her a reason to be reassured.

"In my mind's eye, I saw Rhoda squatting on the floor. But then, she got to her knees, then stood up tall and proud. And she kind of gestured to herself, as if to say, 'See?' That's why she started off crouched on the floor, then stood up – she wanted me to make the connection that it was indeed her spirit I sensed. She tugs on people's legs because that's what they expect to feel from her. She wants people to know it's her. She realizes that people think of her as being blind and crippled.

Happily, that's no longer true. But she also wants people to know that she is whole, healthy and sound now. She feels safe and protected here on the hilltop."

In a later email conversation, Lisa shared some information with me that I found infinitely precious.

"Rhoda is well aware of the fact that you care for her and that she is in your book. You have talked about her right there on the hilltop. She can hear every single word, and it means the world to her."

CHAPTER TWENTY-SIX
RHODA'S LEGACY

How can we possibly say that Rhoda Derry left a legacy? She was blind, she couldn't walk, she didn't speak. Her communication was limited to grunts, gabbling, and the odd yank on a visitor's pants leg. She was no Sojourner Truth, asking "ain't I a woman?" when faced with unfairness. She was no Elizabeth Cady Stanton, no Nellie Bly, no Amelia Bloomer. She didn't even have the writing eloquence of a Helen Keller. So how could she possibly do anything of any lasting consequence?

She survived. It was as simple, and as wrenchingly difficult, as that.

Dr. Zeller was the first to recognize this, but he most certainly wasn't the last. In his letter to the judge of the Adams County Court written when Rhoda died, Dr. Zeller wrote, "Her case alone called down more blessings upon the State than all the eighteen hundred others we are now caring for ... no person ever saw her without becoming a firm convert to the belief in state care of the insane."

Dr. Zeller knew he had an uphill battle to fight, as the superintendent of an insane asylum. I'm sure that when he accepted the invitation from the Peoria Women's Club, he was under no delusion the job would be easy. But it was vitally necessary. The conditions of other institutions for the care of the mentally ill, conditions he saw regularly as he made his inspection rounds as state alienist, taught him that.

He knew that people are visual creatures. Show, don't tell – it's much easier to convince people that way. That was the reason behind the Peoria State Hospital's policy of complete transparency. Inspectors from the asylum's board of trustees came through every several weeks. The staff prided themselves on living up to Dr. Zeller's example.

And Rhoda Derry was Dr. Zeller's poster child. Just by being a patient at the facility, Rhoda was a living, breathing illustration of how much better a state-funded asylum was than the county-run poor farm that had destroyed her life. Even the description of the appalling conditions that had been Rhoda's existence for decades, when placed in contrast to the clean, well-fed patient in front of them, would have captured the attention of any visitor who met Rhoda.

Anyone with $25 and an empty barn could apply for the license to set up an almshouse. There were others, like the almshouses run by each county in Illinois, that had a little more oversight than that. County-run poor houses were meant to provide a place, paid for with county tax money, where poor folks could have a last-ditch place to live. The Adams County Poor Farm was intended to give indigents a place to go. It was not equipped to care for the mentally ill. It's just a sad fact that poor people go crazy too. "They did the best they could" is cold comfort, even at a distance of a hundred and fifty years.

But then, the Peoria Women's Club came up with the idea of establishing an institution specifically for the long-term care of the mentally ill. Ironically, and thankfully, the reason they decided this is because members of the club toured some of these wretched almshouses, and decided they could do better. Dr. Zeller threw his talents behind the idea, and the Peoria State Hospital was born.

The Illinois Asylum for the Incurable Insane, despite its appalling name, was designed expressly to care for the mentally ill on a long-term basis. From the cottage plan, in which patients with similar afflictions were housed together in a sort of "buddy system", to the many forms of therapy available, the entire place was focused on what Dr. Zeller called "that fine old word – asylum". This was a place of refuge, a place where a man wrestling with his demons could put his head down and bull his way through eight hours of work. A place where a deranged woman could retreat to the solace of caring for the vegetables in the cottage garden. A place where the mentally ill could step back from the confusing bustle of life on the outside, take a deep breath, and work on their problems.

Sometimes, though, patients arrived too broken to fix. The asylum had a place for them too.

Nothing anyone can say or write will ever change what Rhoda Derry suffered. Nothing can excuse the atrocity of committing a beautiful, troubled, damaged young woman to an almshouse, then locking her in a crib for decades when she began to self-harm in the depths of her despair. Nothing can justify a life, wasted.

How lucky we are, then, that Rhoda's life, in the end, was not wasted. Thanks to Dr. George Zeller and his staff, we can stand in Cemetery One and look down at the flowers left by Rhoda's admirers, at the white porcelain cherub that keeps silent vigil. We can read the words of quiet sincerity on Rhoda's grave marker.

"They built this place of asylum so that no other human would suffer as you. You taught us to love and feel compassion towards the less fortunate. May you find peace and warmth in God's arms."

And just maybe, as we stand there, we'll feel a sly tug on our pants leg, as the breeze carries to us the faintest whiff of chewing tobacco.

AUTHOR'S NOTE

This is for the readers – and I know you guys are out there, because I'm one of you – who are interested in the process, the back-story, all the sweat and late nights and too many cherry Twizzler bites that go into writing a book.

Ever since 1906, most people's image of Rhoda Derry has been the wizened, withered sack of bones sitting on the floor of Dining Hall A, grinning sightlessly at the camera. But she was so much more than that. She was a young girl in love, a teenager cowed by an imposing figure who had power over her – whether real or imagined. She was a young lady locked away, abandoned by the family who could no longer care for her. I wanted to present Rhoda Derry in all her variety.

When reading a novel, a reader can finish the book with a satisfied sigh and think, "I wonder what happened in their lives after that." Well ... nothing. It's fiction. The characters have no further adventures beyond the page, unless the author writes another book and it turns into a series.

Nonfiction, though, is absolutely the opposite. The characters in a nonfiction book do have lives beyond the covers of the book. They have dreams and hopes and fears and aspirations far beyond the power of an author to describe. They fought, drank, slept, hated, mourned, and loved just as much as we ourselves do.

I've chosen to use some techniques of fiction in this story, describing scenes from Rhoda's and Charles' lives, and from the life of Dr. George Zeller. I did this to give readers a sense of what these people were really like. Too often, characters from the past are just that – stiff, sepia-toned wax models who stand unblinking in old photographs. Their unsmiling faces never betray their humanity, their loves, their hungers, their passions. But they did have passions. They hungered. They loved.

Rhoda and Charles *loved.*

At the same time, I wanted to delve into the social background of the times, to explore what formed the environment in which Charles and Rhoda came of age. As a historian, and as a writer, my biggest and most pressing question is *why?* Why did this love story implode into a tragedy? What expectations shaped Charles and Rhoda? What pressures molded them into the young people who met in 1850 and fell in love? Of necessity, this was a simplified look at the times. I hope, though, that it gave readers a framework of reference on which to place Rhoda's story. Also, I hope it leads to a better understanding of what drove the actors in this drama.

The dialogue used in the first chapter is taken directly from Dr. Zeller's testimony in Washington DC, at the Congressional hearings described. When I read the transcript of these hearings, I could almost hear Dr. Zeller's voice. I had to use his words in the opening chapter – a simple retelling would not have worked half so well.

In February 2014, I spent a few days at my sister's house. She graciously offered me some "peace and quiet" time away from my everyday life – and in fact, that's where this book was born. I had been writing for two days solid when my sister asked me how the new project was going.

Of course I had to tell her Rhoda's story. I spoke fervently about Rhoda's infatuation with Charles, her terror at Nancy Phenix's curse, her decades-long languishing in the Adams County almshouse, Dr. Zeller's compassionate rescue. My sister listened, interrupting once in a while with questions. Doubt laced her tone.

"It all sounds like ... exaggeration. Like someone heard a story back in the day, and blew it all out of proportion, and you're hearing it a hundred and sixty years later and taking it as truth. You can't know what's truth and what's made up at that distance."

She shook her head. "I just think – I think it's wrong to assume that every crazy story you hear about someone is the truth. What probably happened was that someone, a neighbor, said, 'Hey, guess what I heard about Rhoda? I heard she spun around on her head with nothing holding her up.' And knowing how weird she was, because she was mentally ill, people just ran with it."

I do have to admit my sister is extremely sensitive about other people's privacy, whether they are alive or dead, because she is extremely sensitive of her own privacy. (She also regards my ghost hunting as the rudest form of intrusion, something like "upskirt" photos of the dead.) But she's right about this. We can't know which parts of Rhoda's story are true, and which are hearsay handed down through the years. The important part is that she survived her ordeals, and became an inspiration for the care of the mentally ill. And that, I think, is worth a few tall tales.

This was a very emotional book to write. In addition to steeping myself in Rhoda's tragedy for months on end, I made the decision to learn more about my own mother's life, which was no picnic either. I believe there are parallels between the lives of these two women who lived a century apart. I like to think that looking at these parallels added to the story. But I came to realize that devoting a chapter of this book to my beautiful, smart, but damaged mother was not the most intelligent course of action. I wrote that chapter – and indeed, most of this book – at a period in my life when I was battling depression and severe anxiety. I could still function, but only because I didn't have the luxury of curling up and letting the world drift away. I had a book to finish, and a job, and a family to support. Immersing myself in Rhoda's misery, and Dorothy's despair, on top of my own stew of troubles, was not the wisest thing I've ever done.

But I did it anyway. And I think I'm stronger for it.

I'm not the least surprised by my screwy brain. I come from a long and varied line of crazy, including but not limited to suicide, drug addiction, crossdressing, depression, gender confusion, mania, and autism/Asperger's, with some possible schizophrenia thrown in just to flavor the pot. As Augusten Burroughs so eloquently put it in *Lust & Wonder*, "You just cannot mix those raw ingredients together and then stick them inside my mother for nine months and expect something normal to come out."

My sister has little patience with our mother. If Dorothy had lived, I don't know that she and my sister would have had a very good relationship. My sister has said, "I know what it does to *my* brain, to spend time with that complex and needy and self-despising woman. I recoil, even as I have pity."

But I see our mother differently. I see, for better or for worse, a kindred spirit. When Dorothy writes about wanting to hurl something glass against the wall just to experience the shatter, I get that. And I also get why she doesn't do it. I recognize the strength it takes to hold one's shit together.

I recognize how a mind can be so fragile, yet so incredibly strong.

I inherited a lot from my mother – my smile, a love of singing, my habit of dropping a bit of Spanish into my conversations with my dog now and then. And then there are things I inherited from her that are not so innocuous. It's an itch in my brain, a scabrous, snarling black dog slinking around just out of sight. Most of the time, I can ignore it.

I am incredibly grateful for the chance to tell Rhoda Derry's story. Rhoda's life – loving, losing, slipping into insanity, locked away from the world for decades – is an amazing tale, and it deserves to be heard. We are so lucky that Dr. Zeller rescued Rhoda and brought her to the Peoria State Hospital. We are so lucky that Rhoda didn't die in obscurity, that she survived long enough to have her story brought to the world by Dr. Zeller and his staff.

There are so many people who suffer from mental illness. Yes, I'm one of them. And while we don't lock people up in Utica cribs any more, sometimes it can feel like our *minds* are locked away, denied the fresh air and the sunshine that seem to come so effortlessly for every other person on the planet.

But it doesn't *have* to feel that way. There is help. There is hope. (And because I am writing this on a good day, I genuinely believe it.) Seriously, though, it's going to be okay.

And I am not ashamed of what goes on in my head. I sure as hell don't *like* it sometimes. But I'm not ashamed of it. There's no more shame in having mental illness than there is in having diabetes, or COPD, or any other disease. It just happens. And *no one* should be made to feel ashamed of it.

ACKNOWLEDGEMENTS

A book may be written by one person, but there are so many others who help bring it into the world. What you are holding in your hands right now is the hard work of not one person, but many. It's the heart and soul of everyone who helped make this book a reality.

The music that sustained me through this project, especially when writing about the nineteenth century, was music from the era. I especially enjoyed the soundtrack to *Gettysburg: The Boys in Blue and Gray*, with music by Nicholas Palmer. I also found inspiration in *Listen to the Mockingbird*, by The Chestnut Brass Company and Friends, and *"A Tribute to Our Leader"*, by the 33rd Illinois Volunteer Regiment Band.

Huge and totally inadequate bunches of appreciation are due to Chris Morris, Salina Porter, Jackie McDowell, and all the rest of the staff and volunteers at the Peoria State Hospital Museum, the Pollak Hospital, Insane Women Productions, and the Haunted Infirmary. (I think that pretty much covers the conglomeration of all you guys do on the hilltop!) I admire your dedication to the history of the asylum, and your devotion to sharing that history with the next generation.

I appreciate all the staff at the Fondulac Library, for putting up with me while I write, and for asking how things are going. You guys are so wonderful, and I am grateful to spend forty hours a week with you. Thanks to Deb for Swedish Fish, and to Carol for cherry Twizzler bites. We rock Monday evenings!

Thanks to the secretaries and librarians at the historical societies that I bugged over and over in my search for Charles. Thanks most especially to the staff at the Bourbon County and Fort Scott historical society, and to Lin Frederiksen, who tracked down a Charles Phenix for me – not the right one, but a guy with a fascinating story nonetheless.

I stand on the shoulders of giants with every book I write. I'm not sure I would even have attempted this book without the invaluable help of a slim volume entitled *Rhoda: A Tragic and True Story of a Farmer's Daughter*, by D. Doc Derry. This book contained not only the facts of Rhoda's life, but also a wealth of genealogical information compiled by Joan Brown Derry, another family historian. I cannot adequately express my appreciation for the legwork they did long before I even heard of Rhoda Derry. Doc was also extremely gracious in answering my many questions about other members of Rhoda's family.

Another book that inspired me during this project (yes, I read it a couple of times) was *The Sinking of the Eastland*, a nonfiction book by my enormously talented friend Jay Bonansinga, best-selling author of the Walking Dead novels. Jay has always had my back, even when I was just a baby writer. He is genial and kind to young writers, and helpful and encouraging to writers who get a little farther in their journey. In short, he is just the nicest guy you could ever want to meet, and I am so glad to call him my friend.

James Barrow is a fellow paranormal investigator who has a special place in his heart for Rhoda, having had several experiences with her. I thank him profusely for helping me to ask "Why?"

Special thanks are due to my editors, Donelle Whiting and Tracie McBride, and to my publisher, Troy Taylor. Troy, especially, deserves a medal for the patience he showed while we were all pulling this book together.

I have had so much support in writing this book. Many radio show hosts asked me, on behalf of their listeners, to be a guest on their shows. I am grateful to all of them. A special shout-out must go to Jerry Ayres and Jen Kruse of The Calling (Minnesota), for always being such gracious hosts, and insisting that I choose their show to debut *44 Years in Darkness*. I also want to thank Brian and Sherri of The Brian and Sherri Show (New York City), for inviting me onto their show multiple times, and for asking me specifically about the Bowen Building when I was at a particularly low point in working on things. I hope you guys realize now, with this little snippet, how much that meant to me.

To all the people, named and unnamed, who helped me with this book, my deepest gratitude. And to my readers – I hope you enjoy the book we have all crafted for you.

Thank you to my husband, title dreamer extraordinaire, and best friend, Rob. With you, I've found the love of a lifetime. I know I am cherished. That would be wonderful for anyone to know, but with my damaged background, it's precious beyond measure. Thank you for putting up with me, for accepting takeout for dinner too many evenings, and for coming up behind me with shoulder rubs at just the right moments. I love you beyond all reason.

APPENDIX 1:
CHARLES PHENIX

One of the disappointments of working on this book was this: I tried for months to find Charles Phenix. I wanted *so badly* to be the one who turned up evidence of where he had gone after losing Rhoda. I would have settled for finding any members of his family, any Phenixes at all.

After Nancy destroyed Rhoda's life, the family just vanished.

But that's not to say I didn't find *any* Charles Phenixes. I found plenty. You'd be amazed at how common a name it is. I found half a dozen of them all over the United States in the second half of the nineteenth century. One Charles Phenix is even buried in Springdale Cemetery in Peoria, twenty minutes from my house. Some of them I could eliminate right away – they were too young, or too old. One of them was black. There was a Charles W. Phenix who ran a dry goods store in Illinois. There was another Charles Phenix – a young one – who fought in the Spanish-American War, and was killed in March 1900 while raising the flag in Manila. (So yes, there is a possibility, however remote, that Dr. George Zeller knew a Charles Phenix. That ought to make you smile.)

I did follow one Charles fairly far down the rabbit hole. Given the rumor that the Phenixes had moved west, and had possibly ended up in Kansas, I got very excited when I found a Charles H. Phenix in the 1871 city directory of Fort Scott, Kansas, in Bourbon County – a Charles who was also listed in the Bourbon County Marriage Records for 1857-1875. (His birthdate was listed as 1844, but I had my fingers crossed that this was an error in transcription.) He married a Carrie Priest in 1871. I got even more excited when I found an Emaline Phenix with a death date of January 1904. She is buried in Woodlawn Cemetery just outside of Kansas City, Kansas, about an hour north of Fort Scott. (Our Charles had a younger sister named Emaline.) Had I tracked down not one, but two members of the elusive Phenix family?

Had I finally found Charles, after a hundred and fifty years?

I contacted the historical societies in Bourbon County to do more digging. Lin Fredericksen was an invaluable help ... unfortunately, her research confirmed that this Charles Phenix was born to Leander and Mary in 1844, not Frederick and

Nancy in 1834. And Emaline? Who knows? We were unable to find a birthdate for her, or any date other than January 1904.

But what a life this Charles led! Charles Henry Phenix was a landowner who served in the Civil War. He grew up in Peoria, Illinois. He shows up in the 1870 Peoria census with his parents, Leander and Mary. Charles moved away to Kansas very soon after that, and married Caroline (Carrie) M. Priest in 1871 in Bourbon County. He appears in the next census (1880) with Carrie and William Priest, her son from a previous marriage. They lived in Fort Scott for a while, then Charles and Carrie separated. Charles moved to Winfield, Kansas, near Wichita, with his stepson William.

This Charles met an unfortunate end. He was killed over a game of craps.

An article in the *Belleville Telescope* (August 20, 1897), states "In a drunken row over a crap game, Eli Franklin, colored, struck Charles Phenix, white, on the head. Phenix fell on the pavement, receiving injuries from which he died."

And, believe it or not, *that* Charles Phenix is the fellow buried in Springdale Cemetery in Peoria.

APPENDIX 2: GHOST ASYLUM

Rhoda's story is very compelling. People who hear it are at first appalled. *You mean she was caged up for forty-four years?* Then the shock turns to gruesome curiosity. *How could anyone claw their own eyes out?* There are, unfortunately, some people for whom the story ends there. They hear about Rhoda's rescue by Dr. Zeller, but it doesn't really sink in that Rhoda was a real person, with feelings and a history. There are even some ghost hunters that seek out Rhoda just for the ghoulish thrills, and not to show her respect.

In November 2015, I got a phone call from a television producer in California who wanted to talk about Rhoda Derry. (I had done an interview for a local paper the week before, and the reporter had given the producer my information.) The producer and I chatted for a while, then she asked me to show up at the asylum the next week. They were going to film an episode of Ghost Asylum.

Now, I have no problem acting as a consultant for people's projects. I'm happy to share Rhoda's story. But Destination America took the information I gave them, and did absolutely nothing with it. As it turned out, the producers chose not to interview me on camera. It's just as well; the episode was riddled with inaccuracies and outright lies. The "historian" they did have on camera fed the crew the ghoulish asylum stories they were looking for, not any true history.

If you ever watch Season 3, Episode 3 of Ghost Asylum, please know that the whole episode is full of disinformation. The filming makes it look like the Bowen Building ~ what the investigators are calling "the Peoria State Hospital" ~ is the entire asylum. Not true. The Bowen Building is one of thirteen buildings that are left of the asylum. The Bowen was used as a nurses' dormitory and classrooms, not as a venue for bloody experiments. There were never any lobotomies performed in that building.

Neither did they do electroshock therapy in the basement. Why would they do either of those things in a nurses' dorm? The "lobotomy room" on the third floor? Patients' records. That's all. The mesh gate was for protecting the privacy of the records, not for corralling patients. And no one ~ I repeat, no one ~ ever bled out up there. For that matter, no patient at the Peoria State Hospital ever died as the result of a medical experiment. That's a complete lie. The PSH was a place of comfort and of rescue for these patients.

And as far as Rhoda Derry goes, looking seriously for her spirit in the Bowen Building is foolish, as she was never there. She lived for a while in a cottage on C Row, then was moved to Dining Hall A, where she died from tuberculosis. She did not spend her final days "dragging herself around the asylum hallways". She spent her last two years in the care of compassionate nurses, who made sure she got to experience the asylum grounds in any way that was left to her. The nurses let her sit out in the gardens, and feel the sun on her face, and hear birds singing. They took her to dances on Saturday nights, so she could enjoy the music. And building a Utica crib to try and trap her spirit is utterly reprehensible. She spent forty-four years of her life in that hell. It doesn't represent safety ~ it represents decades of desolate horror. Why would she come anywhere near it as a spirit? Trying to trap her, and take her away from the place her spirit found peace, is despicable.

We who know the history of the Peoria State Hospital, and who know Rhoda's story, and who love her, are appalled at the thought of ghost hunters trying to trap her spirit to take her away. I know it's "just a TV show". But it would be just as good for ratings if the crew of Ghost Asylum would show some respect for the people who lived and died at the institutions they investigate.

NOTES

Chapter 2. "So the Illinois Constitution of 1818 protected slavery in some cases, and allowed Southern slave owners to bring blacks into the state for specific purposes." – John Crenshaw took advantage of this when he brought slaves into southern Illinois to work the state- owned salt mines. No free men would perform the arduous labor of the mines, so Crenshaw was granted an exemption. Crenshaw built an empire on the backs of his slaves. He owned thousands of acres of land, in addition to the 30,000 acres he leased from the state for the salt works, and legally owned more than seven hundred slaves. At one time, the taxes he paid amounted to one-seventh the revenue of the entire state. His mansion, later known as the Old Slave House, still stands as a reminder of Crenshaw's ugliness. It was considered a stop on the "reverse Underground Railroad", as Crenshaw would kidnap escaped slaves and free blacks and sell them back into servitude.

Chapter 8. "Valentine Derry, also known as Felty, and Mary Derry, called Moll, were married and living in Germany at the time of the American Revolution." – There are some sources that say that both Valentine and Moll were born in Loudon County , but this is a different branch of the family. For a while, there was speculation that Moll's husband was Jacob, son of Balthazar Derry of Loudon County, Virginia. The Derry family genealogists have since proven that wrong, through DNA testing. Balthazar Derry, otherwise known as Balzer, is related ... they just don't know exactly how.

Chapter 8. "It was thought by [[many]] persons ..." ~ *Mountain Democrat*, Placerville, CA, Saturday, October 25, 1879, page 3. For a complete text of the article, please visit https://sites.google.com/site/derrysinamerica2/maryoldmollderry

Chapter 8. "Moll's oldest son, Bazil Derry, took after both of his parents." – There are a plethora of Basils in the Derry family. Perhaps in homage to his brother, Jacob Derry, Rhoda's father, named his second son Basil. That son went on to name one of his own sons Basil. And Jacob's oldest son, Philip, also named one of his sons Basil.

Chapter 8. "He served for fifteen years, from 1854 to 1869, and his ideas formed the foundation of modern psychiatric care." – Dr. McFarland was brilliant, but like so many of the characters in this book, flawed. (He fits right in.) In September 1862, two years and three months after Elizabeth Packard's arrival, Dr. McFarland was arrested in Springfield and fined three dollars for being "plain dead drunk". And late in 1891, Dr. McFarland realized that he was beginning to suffer from dementia. On November 21, 1891, he committed suicide rather than face a slow decline.

Chapter 11. "The responsibility damaged the girl beyond repair, and she died young, a raving maniac in her thirties." – Elizabeth Packard's only daughter was also named Elizabeth, but called Lizzie or Libbie. When Lizzie was ten, Elizabeth Ware Packard was taken to Jacksonville. The duty of caring for the household fell to Lizzie, who was far too young for this sort of responsibility. After the elder Elizabeth's release, mother and daughter lived for a time with Elizabeth's son Theo, in Pasadena, California. Elizabeth and Lizzie shared the front room of the house, until Lizzie became seriously disturbed. Elizabeth was determined to keep Lizzie out of an asylum, despite the reforms she herself had brought about. Theo built a 10' by 5' enclosure of chicken wire in the front room – just enough space for a cot and a table. Lizzie lived here for months on end, taking her meals on a tray. Eventually, Elizabeth took Lizzie back to Illinois. Shortly after their return to Chicago, Elizabeth died (July 25, 1897). After her death, someone (probably her brother Samuel) did put Lizzie in an asylum. She died there a year later.

Chapter 13. "Levi Slater, Rhoda's nephew, gave a detailed account of her story to the Quincy Daily Journal for an article dated November 23, 1906." – For a complete version of the article, please see D. Doc Derry's book *Rhoda: A Tragic & True Story of a Farmer's Daughter* (Tawana River Publishing, 2011).

Chapter 14. "Another drawback of the Kirkbride system was that all of the patients were housed together." – The first superintendent of the asylum at Kankakee, Richard Dewey, wrote in the 1930s, "In the United States, we had this inflexible plan for all the varying classes of patients, acute and chronic, quiet and disturbed, able-bodied and infirm, alert and impassive, industrious and idle." The Illinois Eastern State Hospital for the Insane, built in 1878 at Kankakee, was designed using a dual system; there was a linear Kirkbride building for housing curable patients, while inmates needing long term care were housed in cottages.

Chapter 15. "In 1874, the city of Quincy reorganized its care of paupers." – The agreement the board came to with the Charitable Aid Association was for the association to keep the overflow of the destitute for ten months, from July 1, 1874 to May 1, 1875, for $8,000 and two hundred cords of wood; and for the next year, beginning May 1, 1875, for a sum not to exceed $12,000. The association managed to do it for $10,400.

Chapter 19. "If you treated a dog like that, you'd be in jail for cruelty." – "One of the coveted bits of political patronage is that of the State Humane Officer but his guardianship does not extend to the human field. The Society for the Prevention of Cruelty to Animals, with all the abuses it has corrected, would have been snubbed had it turned its attention toward the amelioration of conditions surrounding the care of the insane. Had anyone treated a dog or horse as cruelly as were the insane, he would have been speedily brought into court. But the insane had practically no champion outside the asylum and the few voices that were raised in their behalf were stilled with the charge that they were meddlers or ignorant of the problems arising in the daily life of the asylum." Dr. George Zeller, *The Autobiography of George A. Zeller, MD* (Peoria County Genealogical Society, 1995)

Chapter 20. "The new buildings provided living quarters for hundreds more patients." – The employee's building, from the opening of the asylum in 1902 until the construction of the C Row cottages in 1904, was home to 138 criminally insane women, and for very good reason. These were not necessarily violent patients, despite the label "criminally insane". These were simply women who found themselves on the wrong side of the law, in some cases for offenses like stealing bread to feed their children. Some of them were battered women who fought back against their abusers and ended up in jail for it. Dr. Zeller knew that he could not afford to let these women languish in the court system, waiting for their cottage to be built. So he made the decision to house them in the employee's building.

Chapter 20. "In preparation for opening the asylum, the institution arranged to use the railroad spur that ended at the top of the hill." ~ The tracks had been laid decades before, by Sholl Brothers, the coal company that had occupied the hilltop at the end of the nineteenth century. The asylum purchased the track outright from the coal company. In the minutes of the Appropriations for the 50th General Assembly for Illinois, Item 7 reads, "There is hereby appropriated for the Peoria State Hospital for the purchase of Sholl Brothers of the switch track connecting said hospital with the tracks of the Peoria and Pekin Union Railway Company the sum of $35,000, same to be paid upon delivery deed, with a condition that Sholl Brothers may use said track for carrying coal from mines adjoining for a period not exceeding ten years." This appropriation was made in 1917; the coal company and the hospital ended up using the track concurrently for several years.

Interlude. "To add to my mother's stress, my father volunteered his medical services at the Black Panthers' free clinic." ~ Lyndon Johnson started the Child Nutrition Act because the Black Panthers and the Rainbow Coalition were feeding more poor children than the United States government was. (The Rainbow Coalition was a multi-racial alliance between blacks, poor whites, and Puerto Ricans.)

Interlude. "On my mother's death certificate, the cause of death is listed as 'Noludar intoxication, associated hypothermic exposure'." Noludar was withdrawn from the US market in June 1989, in favor of newer drugs with fewer side effects, such as the benzodiazepenes.

BIBLIOGRAPHY

Bartonville – Reports of the Peoria State Hospital.

Bogue, Allan G. *From Prairie to Corn Belt: Farming in the Illinois and Iowa Prairies in the Nineteenth Century* (2nd Edition). Lanham, MD: Ivan R. Dee, 2011.

Clinton, Catherine. *The Other Civil War: American Women in the Nineteenth Century.* New York: Hill and Wang, 1999.

Collins, William H. and Cicero F. Perry. *Past and Present of Adams County.* Chicago: The S. J. Clarke Publishing Company, 1905.

Derry, D. Doc. *Rhoda: A Tragic and True Story of a Farmer's Daughter.* Tawana River Publishing, 2011.

Jacksonville – Reports of the Illinois State Hospital for the Insane, 1847 – 1862. Published Chicago, 1893.

Kriebel, David. *Powwowing Among the Pennsylvania Dutch: A Traditional Medical Practice in the Modern World.* University Park, PA: Pennsylvania State University Press, 2007.

Lowry, Thomas P., MD. *The Story the Soldiers Wouldn't Tell: Sex in the Civil War.* Mechanicsburg, PA: Stackpole Books, 1994.

Pollak, Maxim and Walter H. Baer. *The Friend of the Bereft: George Anthony Zeller, 1858-1938.* Reprinted from *Journal of the History of Medicine and Allied Sciences,* Volume VIII, Number 1.

Portrait and Biographical Record of Adams County, Illinois, containing Biographical Sketches of Prominent and Representative Citizens, together with Biographies and Portraits of all the Presidents of the United States. Chicago: Chapman Bros., 1892.

Quincy and Adams County History and Representative Men (Volume 2). Chicago and New York: Lewis Publishing Company, 1919.

Sapinsley, Barbara. *The Private War of Mrs. Packard.* New York: Paragon House, 1991.

Tillson, Christiana Holmes (Quaife, Milo Milton, ed., with a new introduction by Kay J. Carr). *A Woman's Story of Pioneer Illinois.* Carbondale & Edwardsville: Southern University Press, 1995. (Previously published: Chicago: Lakeside Press, R.R. Donnelley & Sons Co., 1919.)

White, Thomas. *Witches of Pennsylvania: Occult History and Lore.* Charleston: The History Press, 2013.

Ibid. *Ghosts of Southwestern Pennsylvania.* Charleston: Haunted America/History Press, 2010.

Yanni, Carla. *The Architecture of Madness: Insane Asylums in the United States.* Minneapolis: University of Minnesota Press, 2007.

Zeller, Dr. George A. *The Autobiography of George A. Zeller, MD.* Peoria: Peoria County Genealogical Society, 1995.

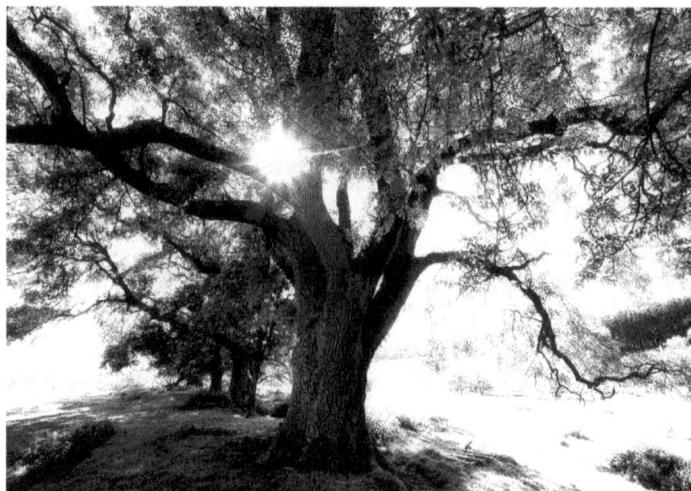

ABOUT THE AUTHOR

Sylvia Shults has been a paranormal investigator for several years, and a historian all her life. She has worked at a library for the past nineteen years, slowly smuggling out enough words in her pockets day by day to build a book of her own. She lives in Illinois with her husband, a certifiably insane Husky fur-daughter, and far too many books. She loves to chat with readers, so please visit her at www.sylviashults.wordpress.com , or on Facebook, on the Fractured Spirits page.

OTHER BOOKS BY SYLVIA SHULTS INCLUDE:

FRACTURED SPIRITS
Hauntings at the Peoria State Hospital

HUNTING DEMONS
A True Story of the Dark Side of the Paranormal

GHOSTS OF THE ILLINOIS RIVER

www.ingramcontent.com/pod-product-compliance
Lightning Source LLC
Chambersburg PA
CBHW071216090426
42736CB00014B/2853